Medicine & Society
In America

Medicine & Society
In America

Advisory Editor

Charles E. Rosenberg
Professor of History
University of Pennsylvania

LETTERS

TO

THE PEOPLE

ON

HEALTH AND HAPPINESS

BY

CATHARINE E. BEECHER

ARNO PRESS & THE NEW YORK TIMES

New York 1972

Reprint Edition 1972 by Arno Press Inc.

LC# 70-180554
ISBN 0-405-03934-4

Medicine and Society in America
ISBN for complete set: 0-405-03930-1
See last pages of this volume for titles.

Manufactured in the United States of America

LETTERS

TO

THE PEOPLE

ON

HEALTH AND HAPPINESS.

BY

CATHARINE E. BEECHER.

NEW YORK:

HARPER & BROTHERS, PUBLISHERS,

FRANKLIN SQUARE.

1855.

INTRODUCTORY NOTICE

THERE are certain portions of this work which the author was unwilling to bring before the public on her own responsibility. With reference to this, proof copies of the work were sent to a large number of cultivated and judicious ladies of influence and position in various sections of the country, in order to secure their opinion as to what should be said and what be omitted.

The result is, there is not a sentence in this work which has not been sanctioned by the approval of those, whom all will concede to be the proper and most highly-qualified judges of propriety on such subjects.

CONTENTS.

PART THIRD.

ABUSES OF THE BODILY ORGANS.

PART FOURTH.

EVILS RESULTING FROM SUCH ABUSES.

PART FIFTH.

REMEDIES FOR THESE EVILS.

NOTES.

LETTERS TO THE PEOPLE

ON

HEALTH AND HAPPINESS.

LETTER FIRST.

My Friends:

Will you let me come to you in your work-shop, or office, or store, or study? and you, my female friends, may I enter your nursery, your parlor, or your kitchen? I have matters of interest to present in which every one of you has a deep personal concern.

I have facts to communicate, that will prove that the American people are pursuing a course, in their own habits and practices, which is destroying health and happiness to an extent that is perfectly appalling. Nay more, I think I shall be able to show, that the majority of parents in this nation are systematically educating the rising generation to be feeble, deformed, homely, sickly, and miserable; as much so as if it were their express aim to commit so monstrous a folly.

I think I can show also, that if a plan for *destroying female health,* in all the ways in which it could be most effectively done, were drawn up, it would be exactly the course which is now pursued by a large portion of this nation, especially in the more wealthy classes.

At the same time, I can present *facts* showing that the results of such a course have been an amount of domestic unhappiness and of individual suffering in all classes in our land that is perfectly frightful, and that these dreadful evils are constantly increasing.

You have read often of the Greeks. Some twenty centuries ago they were a small people, in a small country; and yet they became the wisest and most powerful of all nations, and thus conquered nearly the whole world. And they were remarkable, not only for their wisdom and strength, but for their great beauty, so that the statues they made to resemble their own men and women have, ever since, been regarded as the most perfect forms of human beauty.

The chief reason why they excelled all nations in these respects, was the great care they took in educating their children. They had two kinds of schools—the one to train the minds, and the other to train the bodies of their children. And though they estimated very highly the education of the mind, they still more valued that part of school training which tended to develop and perfect the body.

In the family, too, although the higher classes took care that their children should improve the mind, all, from the highest to the lowest, were earnest in efforts to train the rising generation to have healthy, strong, and beautiful bodies. And when these people met at their national festivals, they not only read or recited history and poetry before these great assemblies, but they still more delighted in games and sports, which exhibited the beauty, strength, gracefulness, and skill of the human body.

But the American people have pursued a very different course. It is true that a large portion of them have provided schools for educating the minds of their children; but instead of providing teachers to train the bodies of their offspring, most of them have not only entirely neglected it, but have done almost every thing they could do to train their children to become feeble, sickly, and ugly. And those, who have not pursued so foolish a course, have taken very little pains to secure the proper education of the body for their offspring during the period of their school life.

In consequence of this dreadful neglect and mismanagement, the children of this country are every year becoming less and less healthful and good-looking. There is a great change in reference to this matter within my memory. When young, I noticed in my travels the children in school-houses, or on Sunday in the churches, almost all of them had rosy cheeks, and looked full of health and spirits. But now, when I notice the children in churches and schools, both in city and country, a great portion of them either have sallow or pale complexions, or look delicate or partially misformed.

When I was young, I did not know of any sickly children. All my brothers and sisters and young playmates could go out in all weathers, were not harmed by wetting their feet, would play on the snow and ice for hours without cloaks or shawls, and never seemed to be troubled with the cold. And the tender parents of these days would be shocked to see how little clothing we wore in the bitterest cold of winter.

But now, though parents take far more pains to wrap up their little ones, to save them from the cold and wet, the children grow less and less healthy every year. And I rarely find a school-room full of such rosy-cheeked, strong, fine-looking children as I used to see thirty years ago.

Every year I hear more and more complaints of the poor health that is so very common among grown people, especially among women. And physicians say, that this is an evil that is constantly increasing, so that they fear, ere long, there will be no healthy women in the country.

At the same time, among all classes of our land, we are constantly hearing of the superior health and activity of our ancestors. Their physical health and strength, and their power of labor and endurance, was altogether beyond any thing witnessed in the present generation.

Travelers, when they go to other countries, especially when they visit England, from whence our ancestors came, are struck with the contrast between the appearance of American women and those of other countries in the matter of health. In this nation, it is rare to see a married woman of thirty or forty, especially in the more wealthy classes, who retains the fullness of person and freshness of complexion that mark good health. But in England, almost all the women are in the full perfection of womanhood at that period of life.

Now it is a fact, that the health of children depends very much on the health of their parents. Feeble and sickly fathers and mothers seldom have strong and healthy children. And when one parent is well and the other sickly, then a part of the children will be sickly and a part healthy.

Thus the more parents become unhealthy the more feeble children will be born. And when these feeble children grow up and become parents, they will have a still more puny and degenerate offspring. So the case will go on, from bad to worse, with every generation. What then, if what I state be true, are the prospects of this nation, unless some great and radical change is effected?

Such a change is possible. The American people have far better advantages than the Greeks had to train their offspring to be strong, healthful, and beautiful, while the means of *retrieving* the mischief already done are in their hands. Nothing is needed but a *full knowledge* of the case, and then the *application of that practical common-sense ana efficiency to this object*, which secures to them such wonderful success in all their business affairs. It is with the hope of doing something to effect such a change that this book has been prepared.

I have been led to this effort by many powerful influences. More than half of the mature years of my own life have been those of restless debility and infirmities, that all would have been saved by the knowledge contained in this work.

More than half the families where I have visited in all parts of the land, seem under a cloud of dim anxiety or sorrow from the failing health or recent death of some beloved member, who has been a victim to similar ignorance.

The many establishments for the restoration of health which I have frequented, are thronged with sufferers from all classes, who bring mournful testimony of the decay of health and vitality in all the circles in which they move, while the statistics of health and disease, which in various ways have been furnished to me, show that the sad impressions made by the above circumstances are more than sustained by unquestionable *facts*. And surely if any thing should "cause the ear that heareth to tingle," it is some of the facts which these pages will present.

All these evils are suffered *chiefly* because the people are ignorant of that which, above all earthly knowledge, they most need to acquire; so that it may truly be said, in the words of Holy Writ—"The people do perish for lack of knowledge."

It is impossible that the evils referred to should be remedied until they are known, and their causes fully understood. And it is impossible to make them comprehended except by giving clear ideas of the construction of certain portions of the human body, the end designed by these organs, and the methods for securing these ends. This is what is first proposed in this work; and in attempting it, the aim will be to avoid all that is not strictly practical, and all the technics of science that are needless. It also will be the aim to write in so clear and simple a style that even children can understand every sentence; and to make the work so *short*, that even American *men of business* can be induced to read it.

The following is an outline of the plan:

The first part contains a brief description of certain organs of the human body most important to health and happiness, and which are most injured and abused by the American people.

The second part shows what is the proper treatment of these organs in order to secure the most perfect health and physical happiness.

The third part points out the various methods in which these organs are most frequently injured.

Part fourth shows the many evil results of such abuse and mismanagement.

Part fifth points out the remedies for these evils.

In regard to the first portion, it is feared that some who are familiar with physiology may pass it over. This is earnestly deprecated. All that follows is so intimately connected with the first part, that none of the work can be fully appreciated after such an omission.

It is a very small book; it will not take over two or three hours to read it.

I beseech you for your own sake, for the sake of all you love best, to read *the whole*.

LETTER SECOND.

In the first place will be given a brief description of certain organs of the human body, the right use of which is most important to health. *The bones* first claim attention as the foundation on which the rest of the body depends for support. There are two hundred and eight bones in the body, besides the teeth. At Fig. 1 and 2 at the end of the book you can see how these bones are arranged and united. The lettering and key show the names of each bone.

The bones are composed of both animal and earthy materials. The animal part gives them life, and the earthy part gives strength. Throw a bone into a fire and the animal part burns out, and what remains is the earthy part, called *lime*. Put a bone into sulphuric acid and water (one part acid and six parts water), and in a few days the acid will remove the earthy part, and what remains will be the soft animal part, which will still retain the shape of the bone.

In infancy the animal part of the bone predominates, and thus children can fall with less danger than grown people, as their bones bend instead of breaking. As age increases, when more caution is gained and more strength is needed, the earthy portion is increased, while in old age it so predominates as to make the bones brittle.

The bones are covered with a thin skin or membrane, filled with small blood-vessels which convey nourishment to them. Where the bones unite with others to form joints, they are covered with *cartilage*, which is a smooth, white, elastic substance. This enables the joints to move smoothly, while its elasticity prevents injuries from sudden jars.

The joints are bound together by strong elastic bands

called *ligaments*, which hold them firmly and prevent dislocation.

Between the ends of the bones that unite to form joints are small sacks or bags, that contain a soft lubricating fluid. This answers the same purpose for the joints as oil in making machinery work smoothly, while the supply is constant, and always in exact proportion to the demand.

The health of the bones depends on the proper nourishment and exercise of the body as much as any part. When a child is feeble and unhealthy, or when it grows up without exercise, the bones do not become firm and hard as they are when the body is healthfully developed by exercise. The size as well as the strength of the bones, to a certain extent, also depend upon exercise and good health.

In this work attention will be directed only to the bones of those parts of the body which are most frequently injured and abused. These are the *thorax*, the *pelvis*, and the *spine*.

The *thorax* is the upper portion of the body, and its bones inclose and protect

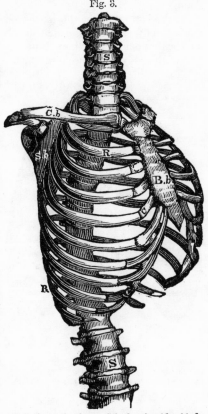

Fig. 8.

C b the collar-bone, S b the shoulder-blade, B b the breast-bone, S the spine, R the ribs.

the heart and lungs.   It consists of the spine or back-bone,
the ribs, the breast-bone, the shoulder-blades and the collar-
bones.   The ribs are fastened to the spine behind, and to
the breast-bone before.   The lower ribs are fastened only
to the spine.   The collar-bones are fastened to the breast-
bone at one end, and at the other end to that point of the
shoulder-blade to which the upper bone of the arm is fastened.   All these bones are bound firmly together by strong
ligaments.

At the bottom of the thorax there is a membrane or skin,
made chiefly of muscles, called the *diaphragm*.   It is in fact
an elastic floor to the thorax, and divides the whole upper
part of the body from the lower part.   The heart and lungs
rest upon it, while the
stomach and liver are
directly under it.   It
is fastened in front to
the breast-bone, be-
hind to the spine, and
at the sides to the
ribs.   It is also fast-
ened in the centre to
the membrane that
separates   the   two
lungs.

Fig. 4.

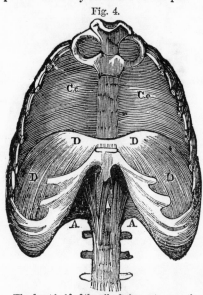

Its muscles are so
contrived that it can
be drawn upward,
thus pressing upward
the heart and lungs.
It also can be drawn
downward, thus pres-
sing the lower in-
testines downward.
Here is a drawing
representing the dia-
phragm in its most
elevated position, the
lungs and heart being
removed.

The front half of the ribs being cut away, the
interior of the chest is exposed.   C c C c the
cavity of the chest, empty.   D D D D the diaphragm, rising high in the centre, and descend-
ing very low at the sides and behind.   The
white space is its tendinous portion.   The
lower part is muscle that contracts to draw it
downward.   A A the abdomen.

When we inspire the air the ribs are drawn upward and outward, making the thorax larger in circumference, and the diaphragm then is drawn down. When we expire the air, the ribs return to their natural place, while the diaphragm is drawn up, as is seen in the previous figure.

As before stated, the lungs and heart rest on the diaphragm, and are moved up and down when it moves, while the liver, stomach, and spleen lie under it.

The thorax is the portion of the body which is habitually *trained to deformity* among American women, as much so as is the foot of a Chinese belle. Every possible method (and there are several) is taken to alter its form, until, in a vast number of cases, it becomes almost inverted in its shape, so that what should be the larger becomes the smaller portion. And there are few women in the more wealthy circles whose

Fig. 5.

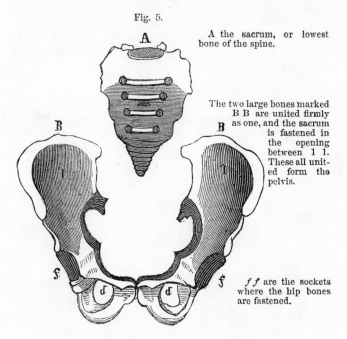

A the sacrum, or lowest bone of the spine.

The two large bones marked B B are united firmly as one, and the sacrum is fastened in the opening between 1 1. These all united form the pelvis.

f f are the sockets where the hip bones are fastened.

thorax is of the proper and natural shape and size. The manner in which this monstrous deformity is produced, and then perpetuated through a degenerate offspring, and the multitudes of diseases and evils that result from it, will be shown in another place.

The lower bones of the body are called the *pelvis*, which are exhibited in Fig. 5.

The middle one is called the *sacrum*, and is the foundation on which the spine rests. The sacrum (A) is inserted in the opening between two large bones, marked B B in the drawing. These bones make the strong foundation on which the body rests when sitting, while the bones of the legs are fastened firmly to it, each side, at *f f*.

The *abdomen* is the portion of the body between the diaphragm and pelvic bones, and contains the organs of digestion and nutrition.

The pelvic organs are the portion of the body the cruel abuses of which have made them the seat of intense and endless suffering to multitudes of both sexes, but especially to American women.

The methods by which this is done will also be pointed out in another part of this book.

A most important portion of the bones, and also one which is strikingly abused, is the *spine*, or *back-bone*. It consists of twenty-four small bones, called vertebræ, piled one above another, and resting on the sacrum, or back part of the pelvis. Here is a drawing of one of the vertebræ.

Fig. 6.

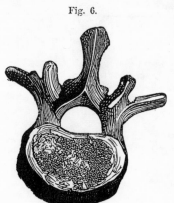

All the vertebral bones have such a hole as is seen in the drawing, and when placed one above another, they so match that the spinal marrow can run through the opening.

Between the vertebræ are placed *cartilage discs*.

These yield to pressure like India rubber, and when the pressure is removed resume their natural form. Here are drawings to illustrate this. Fig. 7 represents two vertebræ; the dark part between them represents the cartilage discs when the spine is in its erect position. Fig. 8 represents the appearance of the disc when the spine is bent forward; and Fig. 9 is the appearance when it is bent backward. The discs yield in the same way when the spine bends to either side.

The bones of the spine are hooked together by a small projection in the upper one sinking into an opening in the lower one, as is shown by a dotted line in Fig. 7. They are also bound together by elastic ligaments, and so strongly, that no bones of the body are so difficult to break or to dislocate as those of the spine.

It is found by measurement, that the pressure of the weight of the

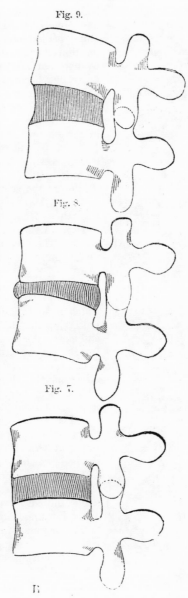

Fig. 9.

Fig. 8.

Fig. 7.

Fig. 10.

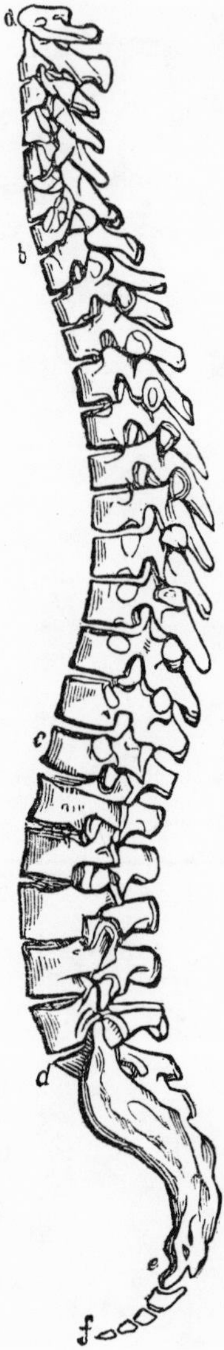

body on the discs of the spine during the day diminishes the height of a person quite perceptibly. But the recumbent position during sleep restores the discs to their natural thickness. In this way, every one becomes a little taller in the morning than at night.

By a back or front view of the spine it is perfectly straight, as may be seen in the view of the whole skeleton, Fig. 1 and 2, at the end of the book. But taking a side view of the spinal column, it is of this form [Fig. 10]. From *a* to *b* are the vertebræ of the neck, from *b* to *c* are those of the back, and from *c* to *d* are those of the loins. From *d* to *e* is the *sacrum*, which is inserted as a part of the *pelvis*. The four little bones at the end finally grow together as a part of the sacrum.

The spine is held in this shape by means of the cartilage discs, each of which is so formed as to do its part in preserving this form. The curving form and elastic discs save the brain and spine from heavy jars, as it thus can gently yield. When the muscles draw the spine in any direction, the elastic discs instantly will restore it to its right form as soon as the force is removed. Thus is curiously contrived a pillar strong enough to hold up the whole body, which yet can bend every way, and while it is itself crooked it holds the body erect.

The spine is held in its position not only by the discs, but by ligaments, by strong muscles, and by the close packing of the intestines against it.

The manner in which this beautiful piece of mechanism is turned to distortion and deformity will be shown hereafter.

LETTER THIRD.

THE bones give strength and form to the body, but the instruments by which it is moved are *the muscles*. They are what in animals is called the flesh, or meat; meaning, not the fat but the red meat.

The muscles are made of very fine threads, called muscular *fibres*, put side by side, and bound up in a thin skin. All these threads are elastic, so that when they are stretched out they shrink back again like India rubber. Here is a drawing that represents the bones of the arm, and of two muscles which we use in bending and straightening it.

All the flesh around the bones of the arm, that make it look plump, is made of layers of muscles, each bound up in a thin case of skin, and fastened strongly to the bones. They are fitted nicely around the bones, the hollow places are filled with fat to give entire roundness, and then the whole is covered with the strong and smooth outer skin. Fig. 12 is a picture of an arm, where all the muscles are shown as

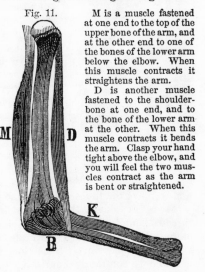

Fig. 11.

M is a muscle fastened at one end to the top of the upper bone of the arm, and at the other end to one of the bones of the lower arm below the elbow. When this muscle contracts it straightens the arm.

D is another muscle fastened to the shoulder-bone at one end, and to the bone of the lower arm at the other. When this muscle contracts it bends the arm. Clasp your hand tight above the elbow, and you will feel the two muscles contract as the arm is bent or straightened.

they appear when the skin is removed. Some of the muscles of the arm are used in turning it, some in lifting it up, some in moving it backward and forward, and some in moving the fingers. Clasp your hand around your arm below the elbow, then shut and open your hand, and you will feel the muscles that move the fingers, some of which open and others shut the hand.

Fig. 12.

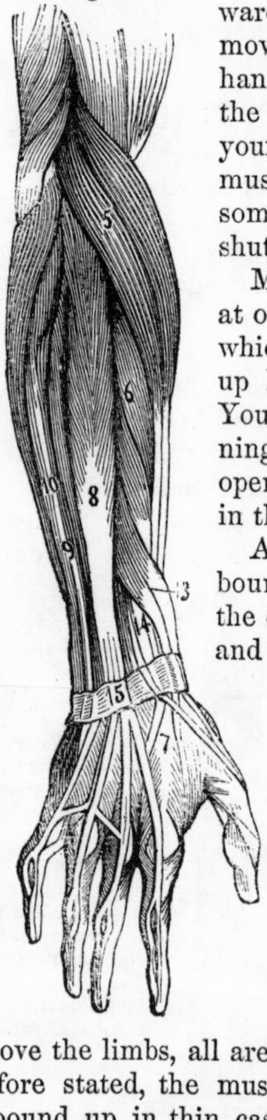

In this drawing the muscles marked 5 and 6 are used in moving the wrist. The one marked 8 extends all the fingers; while another, the other side of the arm, closes them. The one marked 9 moves the little finger; 13 turns the hand sideways, and also moves the arm; 10 and 14 turn the hand; 15 is the strong band that holds the muscles firmly in place around the wrist.

Many of the muscles terminate at one end in cords called *tendons*, which are very strong and take up less room than the muscles. You will see these tendons running across your hand when you open or shut it, and you see them in the drawing.

All the muscles of the body are bound around or lapped one over the others, some being one shape, and some another, according to their uses. There are over five hundred of them; and every movement that is made, either within or without, is accomplished by two or more muscles, one set to draw the part one way, and another set to draw it back again. To swallow the food, to draw the breath, to move the eyes or head, to bend the body and to move the limbs, all are done by the muscles.

As before stated, the muscles are made of fine elastic threads bound up in thin cases of skin. But winding in among these threads are multitudes of little vessels through which the blood flows. This blood is made of the food we eat, and is constantly nourishing every part of the body.

It is brought from the heart by the arteries, and then is carried back to the heart by the veins, as will be explained more at large hereafter.

At present it is only needful to understand how the muscles are nourished by this blood.

Here is a drawing in which is a small artery, *a*, that brings blood from the heart, and then branches out into multitudes of minute blood-vessels. These are called *capillaries*, or *capillary vessels*. They are so small that they can be seen only by very powerful magnifying glasses. This drawing is a magnified view of what in reality is not so large as a pin-head.

Fig. 13.

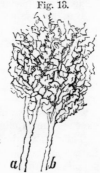

The blood enters these capillaries through the artery, and then meanders through them, depositing its nourishing particles where they are needed, and receiving in return the decayed and useless particles. Then it gradually works its way into the vein, and then the vein carries it back to the heart. Thus the blood is constantly passing from the arteries into the capillaries, and from the capillaries into the veins.

Now every time we move a muscle, some portion of its substance is changed, decays, and is ready to be carried off. At the same time this motion hastens the movement of the blood from the artery which nourishes this muscle, so that it may bring a new supply of nourishment and carry off the dead matter. All exercise of the muscles, therefore, is a process for building up that part of the body exercised with fresh materials. And the more the muscle is exercised, the more close and compact it becomes.

Now the peculiar power of the muscle to *contract strongly*, depends on the firmness and closeness of the muscular fibre. And this firmness can be acquired only by exercise. A muscle that is used but little has but little blood sent to nourish it, and so it becomes pale and soft, and its elasticity or power to contract is diminished. On the contrary, when muscles are well exercised they become firm and compact, have a bright, healthy color, and their contractile power is increased.

The longer and the faster we exercise the muscles the more their firmness and elasticity is increased until they come to the perfect size and shape. If only a few are exercised, then only a small portion of them are strengthened and purified by quicker action. All the rest receive less nourishment, have less life and elastic power, and are consequently imperfectly developed.

But there is a limit to which the exercise of the muscles must be confined, or the excess will be as injurious as a deficiency in exercise. A muscle may be reduced in size, strength, and elasticity by over-exercise; for in this case the decay made by exercise exceeds the supply of nourishment furnished by the blood. This is the reason why horses and oxen that are overworked grow thin and weak. Their muscles are exercised too much, and the decay of muscle exceeds the supply of nourishment furnished by the blood.

This shows the reason, too, why animals must be well fed when they are to be worked hard. The blood must be supplied with more nourishment from food to furnish the supplies needed by the hard-working muscles that are thus constantly decaying and passing away.

But the capillary vessels are not confined to the muscles. The blood nourishes every part of the body, even to the bones, and therefore, every part is supplied with capillaries. There is not a place as large as the point of a needle in our whole body where there are not capillary vessels busily at work in supplying all portions with strength and nourishment.

Exercise not only tends to quicken the movement of the blood in the muscles, but also in all parts of the body. Every portion of the body is decaying and passing away. It is calculated that in about seven years every particle in the body is removed and new matter is supplied instead. Now the more the muscles are used the faster this process proceeds, and the more firmly and purely the body is renewed, provided always the food taken is proper and healthful. Thus the purity and strength of the whole body is dependent on the *proper* exercise of the muscles. If they are exercised too much or too little, debility and emaciation ensue. If they are trained and exercised aright, health, vigor, elasticity, and enjoyment are the result.

LETTER FOURTH.

ORGANS THAT CONVEY THE NOURISHMENT OF THE BODY.

WE have seen the method by which the blood nourishes all parts of the body through the capillaries. We will now attend more particularly to the method by which the blood is carried to and from these capillaries. Fig. 14 is a drawing of the heart as it would look if cut through the middle.

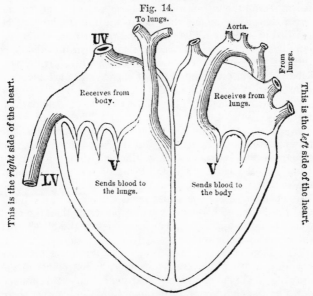

Fig. 14.

The upper right division receives the impure blood from the body through two large veins, marked UV and LV. The lower right division sends the impure blood to the lungs through one large blood-vessel which divides into two, one going to each lung.

The upper left division receives the pure blood from the lungs through three great veins. The lower division sends the pure blood all over the body through the great artery called the *aorta*,

The points marked V show the *valves* through which the blood flows from the upper to the lower divisions of the heart.

In all drawings of the heart it is represented, not as in our own body, but as it would appear to us in another person. Thus the left side of your heart is drawn on the right side of the page, because it represents the heart of a person in front of you.

The left side of the heart contains the pure blood, and the right side holds the impure blood. The upper portions of the heart *receive* the blood from the body and the lungs, and the lower portions *send it out* to the body and the lungs. The impure blood from the body is brought by the veins to the upper right side of the heart, while the pure blood from the lungs enters the upper left side. The impure blood passes from the upper right division of the heart to the lower right division, and then is thrown into the lungs to be purified by the air. The pure blood passes from the upper left division into the lower, and is then thrown into the body through the great artery called the *aorta*, which divides and subdivides almost infinitely as it carries the pure blood to nourish every part of the body.

The heart is made chiefly of very strong muscles, which regularly contract at every pulsation. The upper divisions contract and send the blood into the lower; then the lower divisions contract and send the blood from the right side into the lungs, and from the left side through the aorta into the body. The throbbing of the heart and arteries that we can feel, is made by the contraction of the lower portion of the heart that sends the blood to the lungs and the body. This is much more powerful than the contraction in the upper part, which only sends the blood from the upper to the lower divisions.

The blood passes from the upper to the lower divisions through valves, which are represented by the points in the drawing. These are so made that the blood, as it is pressed down by the contraction of the upper divisions, forces them open. But when the pressure of the blood is the opposite way, as the lower divisions contract, it closes these valves. Thus, when the upper part of the heart contracts, the valves are forced open and the blood passes down; but when the lower divisions contract, the valves are closed tight, and the only place of exit for the blood is through blood-vessels that convey it to the lungs and body.

The aorta also has valves at its junction with the heart, to keep the blood from running back, and the veins all over the body have valves to prevent the blood from running backward when we exercise. This will be explained more clearly at another place.

Here is a drawing which represents the arteries as they divide and subdivide. It is not a very exact drawing of them, but will give a general idea of their course. Those of the head and neck are spread out much more than they are

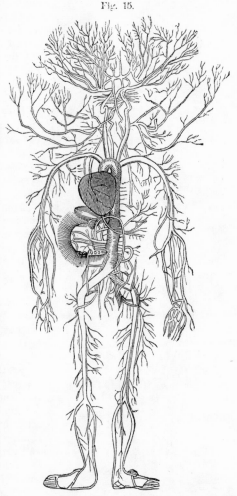

Fig. 15.

in reality, as they could not be easily represented in a drawing any other way. Only the larger arteries are represented. From these branch off thousands of still smaller ones, which

Fig. 16.

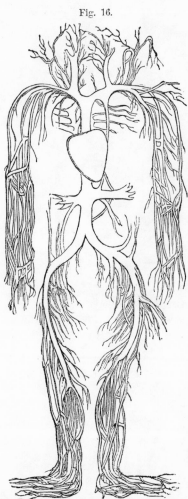

finally terminate in the capillaries. These capillaries can not be represented in this drawing; but turn back to p. 21, Fig. 13, and you will see them. They are at the end of every small vein, and at the end of every small artery, forming a net-work uniting the veins and arteries. The large veins always run very near the large arteries.

From the aorta branch out the arteries to the head and arms above, and to the trunk and legs below. Through these arteries the pure blood from the left side of the heart flows all over the body, to nourish every portion.

Here is a drawing that represents the veins as they carry the blood from the capillaries back to the heart. This also is an imperfect representation, but the large vein coming from the head and arms, and another from the trunk and legs can be seen.

Wherever we find an artery to carry the nourishing blood, near it is a vein to receive it after it has done its office and become impure. The veins are put nearer the surface than the arteries, because it is much less dangerous to cut or injure a vein than an artery.

After the blood has meandered through the capillaries until it has imparted its nourishing parts, and received the decayed portions of the body, it passes through the smallest veins to the larger ones. These carry it to still larger ones, and finally all are united in two great veins, the one coming from the head and arms and the other from the lower parts of the body. Both these great veins empty the impure blood into the right upper portion of the heart.

The pure blood in the arteries is a bright vermilion color. The impure blood in the veins is darker and more of a purple color. The blood in the arteries flows with regular pulsations corresponding with the beats of the heart; but in the veins it flows in a steady stream.

In a full-grown person there are about thirty pounds, or fifteen quarts, of blood, and every beat of the heart sends out about two ounces, while there are from seventy to eighty heart-beats a minute. Thus in each hour over a hogshead of blood passes through the heart. An amount of blood equal to the whole in the body passes through the heart in from six to eight minutes.

In the extremities and capillaries the blood usually flows slower than elsewhere. Thus, though the heart sends out and receives a hogshead of blood every hour, and has an amount *equal* to the blood of the whole body pour through it every six or eight minutes, it is not true that all the blood of the body passes through the heart thus often, for some portions are returned more frequently than others.

Whenever any part of the body is chilled with cold, the blood retreats from that part, and, of course, accumulates in other organs. The health of the body very much depends upon *equalizing the circulation*. It is probable that in a *perfectly* healthy body the circulation is nearly equal in every part.

The manner in which the exercise of the muscles quickens the circulation of the blood will now be explained.

It has been stated that the veins abound in every part of every muscle, and that the large veins have *valves* which allow the blood to pass toward the heart, while they prevent it from flowing the other way.

If the wrist is grasped tightly, the veins of the hand are immediately swollen. This is owing to the fact that the blood is prevented from flowing toward the heart by this pressure, while the arteries, being placed deeper down, are not so compressed, and continue to send the blood into the hand, and thus it accumulates. As soon as this pressure is removed, the blood springs forward from the restraint with accelerated motion. This same process takes place when the muscles are exercised. The contraction of any muscle presses some of the veins, so that the blood can not flow the natural way, while the valves in the veins prevent its flowing backward. Meantime the arteries continue to press the blood along until the veins become swollen. Then, as soon as the muscle ceases its contraction, the blood flows faster from the previous accumulation.

If, then, we use a number of muscles, and use them strongly and quickly, there are so many veins affected in this way as to quicken the whole circulation. The heart re-ceives blood faster, and sends it to the lungs faster. Then the lungs work quicker, to furnish the oxygen required by the greater amount of blood. The blood returns with greater speed to the heart, and the heart sends it out with quicker action through the arteries to the capillaries. In the capillaries, too, the decayed matter is carried off faster, and then the stomach calls for more food to furnish new and pure blood. Thus it is that exercise gives new life and nourishment to every part of the body.

LETTER FIFTH.

WE have seen that the impure blood is sent from the heart to the lungs to be purified. The process by which this is effected will now be explained.

The air we breathe is composed of two invisible gases, called *oxygen* and *nitrogen*. These are always mixed in exactly the same proportions; that is, every hundred pounds of air consists of twenty-one pounds of oxygen and seventy-nine of nitrogen.

There are two other bodies, called *carbon* and *hydrogen;* the first is a solid, and the last a gas. Water is formed by the combination of oxygen and hydrogen gases in certain proportions. If we take away the oxygen from water, what remains is hydrogen, which burns more readily than any other substance.

Carbon is found in wood and coal, which are chiefly composed of it. It is the union of the oxygen of the air with the carbon of wood or coal that produces fire with its light and heat. Almost the whole of our bodies is formed by the combination of *oxygen, hydrogen, carbon,* and *nitrogen.*

The oxygen of the air has a stronger attraction to some bodies than it has to its own nitrogen; so that, in certain circumstances, it will leave the nitrogen, and unite with these bodies. When oxygen unites with carbon, in certain proportions, it forms an invisible gas, called *carbonic acid.* This is heavier than the air, so that, when pure, it can be put in a bowl and poured out like water, and it will then sink to the earth.

Carbonic acid, if taken into the lungs instead of air, will destroy life, though it may be mixed with the air in small quantities, and inhaled without immediate injury. It is

never the case that the air is perfectly free from a small
quantity of this gas.

Having explained the construction of the air, we will now
notice that of the lungs.   Here is a drawing (Fig. 14)
which represents the *windpipe* (or *trachea*) and the *bron-*

Fig. 14.

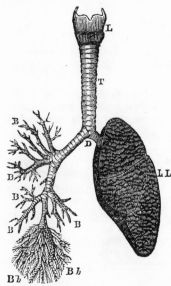

L larynx, or top of the windpipe.

T windpipe.

D two branches of the windpipe.

B, B *b* branches of the windpipe inside of the lungs.

L L outside of one lung.

chial tubes, which convey air to the lungs, and are branches of
the windpipe.   These branch out into innumerably fine tubes,
each one of which terminates in an air-cell.   In this drawing
you see the outside of one of the lungs on the right hand,
and on the other side you see the branches of the windpipe.

On the next page is an enlarged view of the air-cells
which are at the end of the air-tubes that run from the
windpipe.   Fig. 15 shows them as cut open, and Fig. 16
presents the outside of them.   These air-cells are formed
chiefly of capillaries, which receive the blood sent from the
heart to the lungs.   Thus when the air-cell is filled with the

Fig. 15.   Fig. 16.

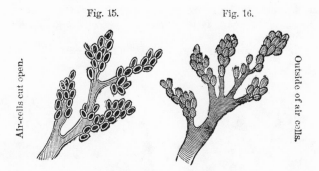

Air-cells cut open.

Outside of air cells.

air we breathe, it at the same time has its capillaries filled with blood. Thus the air and the blood have nothing but a very thin skin, or membrane, to separate them.

Fig. 17.

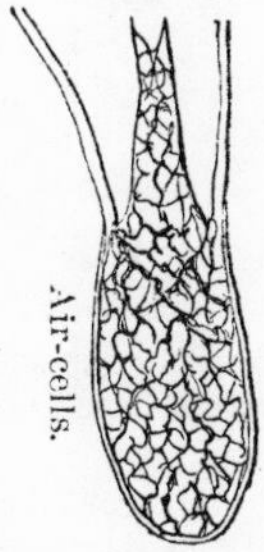

Here is a drawing (see Fig. 17) that represents an enlarged air-cell. It shows how the blood is brought by an artery to the air-cell, and then, after winding through the capillaries, how it flows to the vein which conducts it back to the heart.

Vein. Branch of the windpipe. Artery.

Air-cells.

Now, it is while the blood is thus passing through these capillaries of the air-cells that the process of its purification takes place. The impure part of the blood consists chiefly of *carbonic acid*. This acid has a stronger attraction for the air in the cell than for the blood, and so it passes through the thin membrane and unites with the air. At the same time the oxygen of the air has a stronger attraction for the blood than it has for its own nitrogen, and so it also passes through the membrane and joins the blood in the capillaries.

Thus the blood in the capillaries of the air-cells is purified by giving up its carbonic acid to the air, and receiving the oxygen of the air in return. The air expired from our lungs has thus lost a large portion of its oxygen, and received as much carbonic acid in its place.

When the blood comes into the capillaries of the air-cells,

it is impure with carbonic acid; when it returns from the lungs to the heart, it is supplied with the life-giving and purifying oxygen.

Here is a drawing (Fig. 18) showing the heart with parts

Fig. 18.

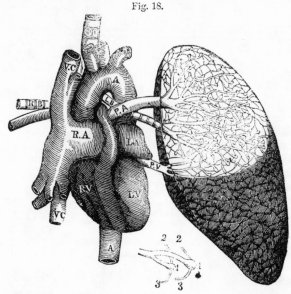

A aorta. T windpipe. L B left branch of the windpipe. P A artery carrying blood to the lungs. P V vein bringing blood back to the heart.

of its great veins and arteries, and also one of the lungs. The upper part of the lung is divested of its external part, to show the manner in which the arteries and veins carry the blood to and from the heart. The one, marked P A, takes the blood to the capillaries of the air-cells, the other, marked P V, brings it back to the heart, while a branch of the windpipe, marked L B, conveys air to the air-cells.

We will now attend to another process which takes place in the capillaries all over the body. We have seen how the blood is carried by the arteries to nourish the whole body. This blood has been furnished with *chyle* by the stomach, and with oxygen by the lungs. As it passes through the capillaries of the body the oxygen is attracted by the carbon of the decayed portions which need to be removed. This union of the oxygen and carbon produces the carbonic acid which renders the blood dark and impure. The veins collect this impure blood and carry it to the heart. At the same time the fresh chyle is deposited in place of the decayed matter, which has been thus removed.

We shall see, in another place, that this union of the oxygen and carbon in the capillaries produces the animal heat which keeps our bodies warmer than the air around us.

The great thing, then, which is indispensable to the purifying of the body is, that the lungs should have a full supply of oxygen. There are two ways in which this is prevented: one is, by the mixture of carbonic acid with the pure air, and the other is, by thinning the air with heat.

We should take about half a pint of air at each inspiration. Now, if a large portion of this is carbonic acid, instead of the pure atmosphere, we lose the same proportion of the needful supply of oxygen at every breath. Heat makes the air thinner, so that there is less oxygen in half a pint of warm air than in the same quantity of cold air. If we breathe warm air, then, less oxygen is obtained than when we breathe cold air.

We have seen how the air is thrown out from the lungs, loaded with carbonic acid, and deprived of its oxygen. As we breathe about twenty times a minute, and use half a pint of air at each breath, it can be seen by calculation that every pair of lungs vitiates one *hogshead* of air every hour. For this reason, it is indispensable to the health of the body that, when we are confined to any room, there should be a gentle but constant current, that shall carry off every hour just as much air as the lungs in that room have vitiated. This is the guide to the rule for ventilating rooms. Just in proportion to the number of persons breathing in a room or house, should be the amount of air brought in and carried out by the arrangements for ventilation.

The membrane that forms the air-cells of the lungs, if all united and spread out in one sheet, would cover the floor of a room twelve feet square. Every breath that fills the lungs brings a surface of air of this size in contact with this extent of membrane, and then the oxygen of the air and the carbonic acid of the blood change places. This shows more vividly what mischief must ensue when the air thus inspired is loaded with carbonic acid from other lungs, in place of the pure and life-giving oxygen.

Every hundred pounds of pure air taken into the lungs, returns with eight pounds of carbonic acid in place of the oxygen given up to the blood.

The air can not retain over ten per cent. of carbonic acid. After thus much has been mixed with the air no more can be received. Were it not for this the air would be oftener rendered entirely deadly, so that life would cease in great crowds.

There are two methods by which the lungs are filled with air; one is, by a rising and outward motion of the ribs enlarging the space around the lungs. Then the air rushes in and fills the air-vessels in the upper portion of the lungs.

The other method is, by the action of the diaphragm and abdominal muscles. The diaphragm, by the contraction of its muscles, is drawn downward, and thus the intestines are pressed downward. This enlarges the space at the bottom of the lungs, and the air fills the air-cells in that portion. Then the muscles of the abdomen contract, and press the intestines upward against the diaphragm, which also moves upward. In this way the air is expelled from the lower portion of the lungs.

There are more air-cells in the lower than in the upper part of the lungs, and for this reason the abdominal breathing is of more consequence than the breathing effected by the ribs.

When the body is perfectly free, and breathing natural, there is more motion of the abdomen than of the chest in breathing. This may be observed in a healthy young child.

It is important that this should be well understood, as the modes of dress are often such as to stop the abdominal breathing almost entirely, and thus to keep a large portion of the lower cells of the lungs entirely without air.

LETTER SIXTH.

WE have seen how the blood is carried by the arteries from the heart into the capillaries, and that the whole body is nourished by it in these minute vessels.

We will now attend to the process by which the blood is manufactured from the food and drink. The solid portions of food are first divided by chewing, in order to mix it with the *saliva* or spittle. This liquid exudes from small *glands* or bags placed near the sides of the mouth. Its use is to moisten the food, so that it will glide easily down to the stomach, and it also aids in dissolving it.

The stomach is a bag that will hold from a quart to three pints, according to the size and age of a person. Here is a drawing showing its shape. It has an inner skin, which

Fig. 19.

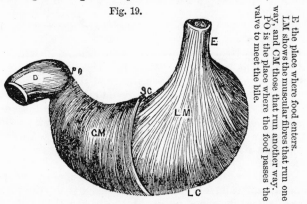

E the place where food enters. LM shows the muscular fibres that run one way, and CM those that run another way. PO is the place where the food passes the valve to meet the bile.

consists chiefly of blood-vessels, from which exudes the *gastric juice* furnished by the blood to dissolve the food. The blood-vessels in this inner skin also draw into the blood all water or other liquid that enters the stomach, except what may be needed to keep the food of a proper consistency during the process of digestion.

The middle coat of the stomach consists chiefly of mus-cles, one set running across and the other set lengthwise. In the drawing the outer skin is removed in one portion to show the muscles.

As soon as food enters the stomach, these muscles begin to contract and relax alternately; making a motion that turns the food over and over, and moves it constantly from one end of the stomach to the other, in order that it may be thoroughly mixed with the gastric juice. The outer skin of the stomach is a smooth and strong covering for the whole, which protects the laboring muscles from injury.

After the food enters the stomach, the veins of the inner skin draw off the superfluous liquids, and then the gastric juice pours into the stomach, and the muscles work with strong and steady action, from two to four hours, until the food is reduced to a thin paste. It then passes through a small *valve*, or door, which opens at the smaller end of the stomach to whatever food is well prepared; but if any comes that is still undigested, this valve closes tight and the food returns till it is properly digested. Should there be food that will not digest, it keeps returning to this valve till its muscles are tired out, and then the undigested mass is al-lowed to pass through.

After passing this valve (which is marked PO in the drawing) the food receives *bile* from the *liver*, and also the *pancreatic juice* from the *pancreas*, and these two liquids change it into a thinner, whitish liquid called *chyle;* then it passes through the lower intestines. Fig. 20 (on the next page) is a drawing of the organs described, together with the lower intestines, through which the chyle is carried. They are not in their natural position, as they are when packed closely in the body.

The chyle, when prepared, passes through the white, smooth, satin-like intestines, that are about twenty-four feet long, all neatly folded up in the body. On the inside of these intestines are the mouths of very small tubes, called *lacteals*, about the size of a fine hair, which gradually draw off this chyle and carry it to a reservoir called the *thoracic*

Fig. 20.

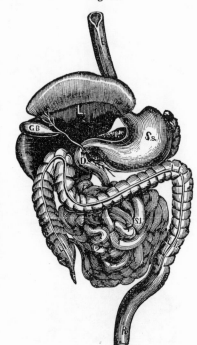

L is the liver.

S s is the stomach.

P is the pancreas, most of it hid.

G B is the gall-bladder that receives the bile.

S is the spleen, most of it hid.

D is the place where the bile and pancreatic juice enter.

S I are the small intestines through which the chyle passes.

L I is the colon, or large intestine, and at its end is the *rectum*, marked R, which is the outlet.

duct. This empties it into a vein near the heart, to be mixed with the other blood.

Fig. 21 (on the next page) is a picture of a small portion of the intestines, with the little vessels drawing off the chyle, and carrying it to the throracic duct. It should be examined by aid of the key at the bottom of the page before proceeding.

It has been shown that the body is constantly decaying, and its dead particles are carried away by the veins, while the arteries bring a new supply of fresh blood from the heart to the capillaries. It is here shown how the capillaries are all depending on the stomach to furnish them with fresh chyle, which is to supply the place of the particles removed.

Fig. 21.

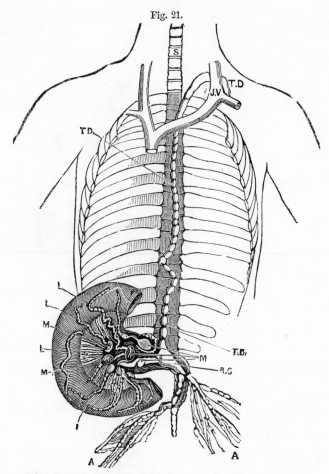

S the windpipe.

T D the thoracic duct.

J V jugular vein into which the thoracic duct empties the chyle.

R C a reservoir that receives the chyle from the intestines.

L M a portion of the smaller intestines where the *lacteals* are seen drawing the chyle and carrying it to the reservoir R C.

A A are lacteals coming from other parts of the intestines with chyle to be emptied into the reservoir R C.

The stomach is so made that as soon as the capillaries need more chyle the sensation of *hunger* comes.   This is the call of the stomach for more food, and if the needful supply is not obtained, a feeling of weakness and faintness pervades the whole body.   Every part is calling for its needed food, and if it is withheld very long the suffering becomes intolerable.   There is no suffering more distressing than this pining of every part of the body for the nourishing particles that the capillaries receive from the chyle, which the stomach alone can supply.

One of the most important portions of this subject is the manner in which the intestines in the thorax and abdomen are *packed* and retained firmly in their right position through all the labors, accidents, and injuries to which the body is exposed.

It has been shown that the thorax is filled with the heart and lungs.   The foundation or elastic floor on which they rest is the diaphragm, whose muscles, by contracting and relaxing, lift the heart and lungs upward when we expire, while they sink when we inspire the air.

Directly under the diaphragm are the stomach, liver, spleen, and pancreas.   Under these are the long intestines through which the chyle passes; and beneath the whole are the pelvic organs.

Fig. 22 (on the next page) and its key illustrate the position of these organs, and should be examined here.

In the front outer covering of the abdomen are very important muscles which press the intestines firmly *inward* and *upward*.   These are called the *abdominal muscles*.   Some run across the abdomen from side to side, and are fastened to the hips and ribs.   Some run upward and downward, and are fastened above to the breast-bone, and below to the pelvic bone.   Besides holding up the intestines in their place, these muscles have a most important office in aiding respiration.   When the diaphragm contracts it is drawn downward, and thus presses the abdominal viscera downward. This makes room for air in the lungs, which rushes in and fills the lowest air-cells.   Then the diaphragm relaxes, and the abdominal muscles contract, pressing the intestines upward, and thus pressing the air out of the lungs.

Fig. 22.

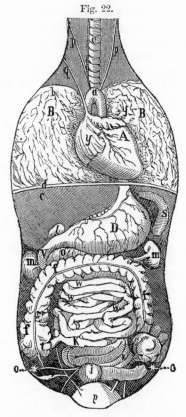

Packing of the intestines.

c the windpipe.
a the aorta.
A the heart.
B B the two lungs.
d the diaphragm at its lowest position when the lungs
are inflated.
c the liver.
D the stomach.
S the spleen.
l the gall-bladder.
o the pancreas.
m m the two kidneys.
w w the smaller intestines
through which the chyle first
passes.
f f the *colon*, or largest intestine, that terminates with
the rectum, which is the final
exit from the body.
o o the two ovaries ⎫
i the uterus. ⎬ pelvic
p the bladder. ⎭ organs.

    This alternate pressing of the diaphragm downward, and then of the abdominal muscles upward, is the process of *abdominal respiration.*

    Some of the most dreadful evils that afflict both sexes re-sult from a debility and relaxation of the abdominal muscles, which lessen their power to sustain the intestines that de-pend on them for support. In consequence of this there are displacements and disordered action that inflict the most terrible suffering, especially on the female sex. The evils from this cause will be explained hereafter.

LETTER SEVENTH.

THE body has no power to move itself, but is a collection of instruments to be used by the mind in securing various kinds of knowledge and enjoyment. The organs through which the mind controls all the other portions of the body are the *brain* and *nerves*.

The drawing on the next page (Fig. 23) represents them. The brain lies in the skull, and is divided into the large or upper brain, and the small or lower brain. From the brain runs the spinal marrow through the spine or backbone. From each side of the spine the large nerves run out into innumerable smaller branches to every portion of the body. The drawing shows only some of the larger branches.

The brain and nerves consist of two kinds of nervous matter; the *gray*, which is supposed to be the portion that originates and controls a nervous fluid which imparts power of action; and the *white*, which seems to conduct this fluid to every part of the body.

The brain and nervous system are divided into distinct portions, each having different offices to perform, and each acting independently of the others. One portion is employed by the mind in thinking, in feeling pleasurable or painful emotions, and in choosing or willing. The nerves that run to the nose, ears, eyes, and tongue, are employed in seeing, hearing, smelling, and tasting.

The *back* portion of the spinal marrow and the nerves that run from it are employed in *sensation*, or the *sense of feeling*. These nerves extend over the whole body, but are largely developed in the net-work of nerves in the skin. The *front* portion of the spinal marrow and its branches are employed in moving the muscles in all parts of the body that are controlled by the *will* or *choice* of the mind. These are called the *nerves of motion*.

The nerves of sensation and nerves of motion, although

Fig. 23.

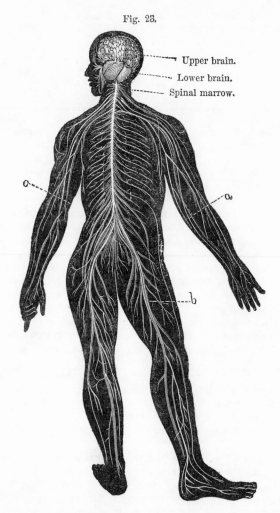

Upper brain.
Lower brain.
Spinal marrow.

they start from different portions of the spine, are united in
the same *sheath*, or *cover*, in most of their branches.   Thus,
every muscle is moved by **nerves of motion**, while alongside
of this nerve, in the same sheath, is a nerve of sensation.

All the nerves of motion and sensation are connected with that part of the brain that thinks, feels, and chooses, and this is supposed to be the seat of the mind. By this arrangement the mind *knows* what is wanted in all parts of the body by means of the nerves of sensation, and then it *acts* by means of the nerves of motion. For example, when we feel the cold air on the skin, the nerves of sensation report to the brain, and thus to the mind, that the body is growing cold. The mind thus knows that more clothing is needed, and *wills* to have the eyes look for it, and the hands and feet move to get it. This is done by the nerves of sight and of motion.

Next are the nerves of involuntary motion, which move all those parts of the head, face, and body, that are used in breathing, and in other operations connected with it. By these we contrive to breathe when asleep, and whether we will to do so or not. There are also some of the nerves of voluntary motion that are mixed with these, which enable the mind to stop respiration, or to regulate it to a certain extent. But the mind has no power to stop it for any great length of time.

There is another large and important system of nerves called the *sympathetic* or *ganglionic* system. It consists of small masses of gray and white nervous matter, that seem to be small brains with nerves running from them. These are called *ganglia*, and are arranged each side of the spine, while small nerves from the spinal marrow run into them, thus uniting the sympathetic system with the nerves of the spine. These ganglia are also distributed around in various parts of the interior of the body, especially in the intestines, and all the different ganglia are connected with each other by nerves, thus making one system.

It is this portion of the nervous system that carries on the circulation of the blood, the action of the capillaries, lymphatics, arteries, and veins, together with the work of secretion, absorption, and most of the internal working of the body, which goes forward without any knowledge or control of the mind.

The following is a recapitulation of the preceding divisions of the nervous system :

First, the brain, which thinks, wills, and feels pleasurable or painful emotions.

Second, the nerves of seeing, hearing, tasting, and smelling.

Third, the nerves of respiration and the operations connected with it.

Fourth, the nerves of sensation and of motion united.

Fifth, the ganglionic or sympathetic nerves.

There are a few nerves not included in this classification, but there is no need of describing them.

Every portion of the body has nerves of sensation coming from the spine, and also branches of the sympathetic or ganglionic system. The object of this is to form a sympathetic communication between the several parts of the body, and also to enable the mind to receive through the brain some general knowledge of the state of the whole system. It is owing to this that when one portion of the body is diseased, other portions sympathize. For example, if one part of the body is diseased, the stomach may so sympathize as to lose all appetite until the disease is removed.

All the operations of the nervous system are performed by the influence of the nervous fluid, which is generated in the gray portions of the brain and ganglia. Whenever a nerve is cut off from its connection with these nervous centres, its power is gone, and the part to which it ministered becomes lifeless and incapable of motion.

The brain and nerves can be overworked, and can also suffer for want of exercise, just as the muscles do. It is necessary for the perfect health of the brain and nerves that the several portions be exercised sufficiently, and that no part be exhausted by over-action. For example, the nerves of sensation may be very much exercised, and the nerves of motion have but little exercise. In this case, one will be weakened by excess of exercise, and the other by the want of it. It is found by experience that the proper exercise of the nerves of motion tends to reduce any extreme susceptibility of the nerves of sensation. On the contrary, the neglect of such exercise leads to produce an excessive sensibility in the nerves of sensation.

Whenever that part of the brain which is employed in thinking, feeling, and willing, is greatly exercised by hard study, or by excessive care or emotion, the blood tends to the brain to supply it with increased nourishment, just as it flows to the muscles when they are exercised.   Over-exercise of this portion of the brain causes engorgement of the blood-vessels.   This is sometimes indicated by pain, or by a sense of fullness in the head; but oftener the result is a debilitating drain on the nervous system, which depends for its supply on the healthful state of the brain.

The brain has, as it were, a fountain of supply for the nervous fluid, which flows to all the nerves, and stimulates them to action.   Some brains have a larger, and some a smaller fountain, so that a degree of mental activity that would entirely exhaust one, would make only a small and healthful drain upon another.

The excessive use of certain portions of the brain tends to withdraw the nervous energy from other portions, so that one part is debilitated by excess, and the other by neglect. For example, a person may so exhaust the brain power in the excessive use of the nerves of motion by hard work, as to leave little for any other faculty.   On the other hand, the nerves of feeling and thinking may be so used as to withdraw the nervous fluid from the nerves of motion, and thus debilitate the muscles.

Some animal propensities may be indulged to such excess as to produce a constant tendency of the blood to a certain portion of the brain, and to the organs connected with it, and thus cause a constant and excessive excitement, which finally becomes a disease.   Sometimes a paralysis of this portion of the brain results from such an entire exhaustion of the nervous fountain and of the overworked nerves.

So, also, the thinking portion of the brain may be so overworked as to drain the nervous fluid from other portions that thus are debilitated by the loss.   And in this way, also, the overworked portion may be diseased or paralyzed by the excess.

The importance of the *equal development* of all portions of the brain by an appropriate exercise of *all* the faculties of mind and body, and the influence of this upon happiness is the most important portion of this subject, and will be more directly exhibited in another letter.

LETTER EIGHTH.

WE have seen that the lungs provide the oxygen for the capillaries, and also throw out the decayed particles of the body, as it day by day is decomposed and passes away. But this labor of purifying is not done by the lungs alone; the kidneys, lower intestines, and skin, all aid, while the skin does more than any other organ. Experiments prove that of every *eight* pounds of food and drink taken, *five* pass off through the skin.

There is no part of the body that is so complicated with curious and wonderful contrivances as the skin; nor is there any that is so effective in causing either good or bad health. It consists of two layers: the outside skin, called the *cuticle*, which is very thin; and the under skin, which is much thicker, called the *true skin*.

The cuticle is at first a transparent fluid that exudes from the blood-vessels of the skin, is spread over the true skin, and becomes hardened into a thin layer. The cuticle is constantly forming and passing away. The external part, by evaporation, changes into thin, dry scales which rub or drop away, while the blood constantly renews the under portion. The white, scurfy substance that passes off so distinctly in taking a warm bath, is the refuse portion of the cuticle. It is the under portion of the cuticle that gives color to all complexions, and which appears so diversely in the European and African races. The cuticle serves to protect the delicate texture of the true skin from injury.

The true skin consists chiefly of a net-work of blood-vessels, nerves, lymphatics, oil glands, and perspiration tubes; while on the head and several other parts of the body hair is also embedded and nourished in the skin. Fig. 24 is a drawing

Fig. 24.

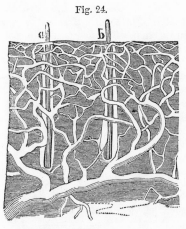

which represents some of the blood-vessels of the skin, and two hairs. It is very greatly magnified. In all parts of the skin are capillaries with small arteries that bring the blood to them, and small veins that carry it back to the heart. The blood thus meandering through the capillaries of the skin, exceeds in quantity what is contained in all the other capillaries of the whole body.

Here is a drawing, greatly magnified, which shows the

Fig. 25.

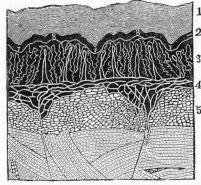

1   1 is the cuticle.

2   2 is the colored part of it.

3   3 and 4 show the network of nerves in the true skin.

4

5   5 is the lower portion of the true skin, showing two points where two nerves from the spinal marrow enter and spread out into the net-work above.

manner in which the nerves are spread through the true skin. The nerves and capillaries interlace; and so minute and close are they, that the point of a needle can not touch any point in the skin without touching both a nerve and a blood-vessel.

Fig. 26 is a drawing that represents a greatly magni-

fied view of the *lymphatics* or *absorbents*. These are ex-
tremely minute vessels that interlace with the nerves and
blood-vessels of the skin. Their office is to aid in collecting the useless, injurious, or decayed matter, and carry
it to certain reservoirs, from which it passes into some of
the large veins to be thrown out through the lungs, bowels,
kidneys, or skin. These
absorbent or *lymphatic ves-*
sels have mouths opening
on the surface of the true
skin, and though covered
by the cuticle, they can absorb both liquids and sol-
ids that are placed in close
contact with the skin. In
proof of this, one of the
main trunks of the lym-
phatics in the hand can
be cut off from all com-
munication with other portions, and tied up. Then
if the hand is immersed in milk a given time, it will be·
found that the milk has been absorbed through· the cuticle, and fills the lymphatics. In this way long-continued
blisters on the skin will introduce the blistering matter
into the blood through the absorbents, and then the kidneys
will take it up from the blood passing through them to carry
it out of the body, and thus become irritated and inflamed
by it.

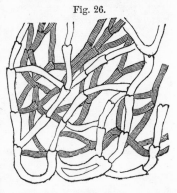

Fig. 26.

There are also oil tubes imbedded in the skin that draw
off oil from the blood. This issues on the surface and
spreads over the cuticle to keep it soft and moist.

But the most curious part of the skin is the innumerable
minute perspiration tubes. Fig. 27, on the opposite page,
is a drawing of one very greatly magnified. These tubes
open on the cuticle, and the openings are called *pores* of the
skin. They descend into the true skin, and then form a
coil, as seen in the drawing. These tubes are hollow, like
a pipe-stem, and their inner surface consists of wonderfully-
minute capillaries filled with the impure venous blood. And

in these small tubes the same process is going on as takes place when the carbonic acid and water of the blood is exhaled from the lungs. The capillaries of these tubes through the whole skin of the body are thus constantly exhaling the noxious and decayed particles of the body, just as the lungs pour them out through the mouth and nose. It is calculated that about three or four pounds of waste matter pass off through the skin every twenty-four hours, and chiefly in the form of carbonic acid and water.

It has been shown that the perspiration tubes are coiled up into a ball at their base. The number and extent of these tubes are astonishing. In a square inch on the palm of the hand have been counted, through a microscope, thirty-five hundred of these

Fig. 27.

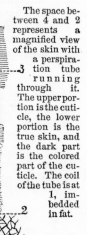

The space between 4 and 2 represents a magnified view of the skin with a perspiration tube running through it. The upper portion is the cuticle, the lower portion is the true skin, and the dark part is the colored part of the cuticle. The coil of the tube is at 1, imbedded in fat.

tubes. Each one of them is about a quarter of an inch in length, including its coils. This makes the united lengths of these little tubes to be seventy-three feet to a square inch. Their united length over the whole body is thus calculated to be equal to *twenty-eight miles!* What a wonderful apparatus this! And what mischiefs must ensue when the *drainage* from the body of such an extent as this becomes obstructed?

But the inside of the body also has a skin, as have all its organs. The interior of the head, the throat, the gullet, the lungs, the stomach, and all the intestines are lined with a skin. This is called the *mucous membrane,* because it is constantly secreting from the blood a slimy substance called *mucus.* When it accumulates in the lungs it is called *phlegm.* This inner skin also has nerves, blood-vessels, and lymphatics. The outer skin joins to the in-

D

ner at the mouth, the nose, and other openings of the
body, and there is a constant sympathy between the two
skins, and thus between the inner organs and the surface
of the body.

The skin has the office of regulating the heat of the body
by a process that will be explained in another place.

SECRETING ORGANS.

Those vessels of the body which draw off certain portions
of the blood and change it into a new form, to be employed
for service or to be thrown out of the body, are called *secreting organs.* The skin in this sense is a secreting organ, as
its perspiration tubes secrete the bad portions of the blood
and send them off.

Of the internal secreting organs the liver is the largest.
Its office is to secrete from the blood any excess of carbon.
For this purpose a set of veins carry the blood of all the
lower intestines to the liver, where the excess of carbon is
drawn off in the form of *bile,* and accumulated in a reservoir called the *gall-bladder.* From thence it passes to the
place where the smaller intestines receive the food from the
stomach, and there it mixes with this food, and aids in preparing it for use. Then it passes through the long intestines, and is thrown out of the body through the rectum.
The liver also has arterial blood sent to nourish it, and corresponding veins to return this blood to the heart. So there
are two sets of blood-vessels for the liver, one to secrete the
bile, and the other to nourish the organ itself.

The kidneys secrete from the arteries that pass through
them all excess of water in the blood, and certain injurious
substances. These are carried through small tubes to the
bladder, and thence thrown out of the body.

The *pancreas* secretes from the arteries that pass through
it the pancreatic juice, which unites with the bile from the
liver in preparing the food for nourishing the body.

There are certain little glands near the eyes that secrete
the tears, and others near the mouth that secrete the saliva
or spittle.

These organs all have arteries sent to them to nourish
them, and also veins to carry away the impure blood. At

the same time they secrete from the arterial blood the peculiar fluid which it is their office to supply.

All the food that passes through the lower intestines which is not drawn off by the lacteals or by some of these secreting organs passes from the body through a passage called the *rectum*.

Learned men have made very curious experiments to ascertain how much the several organs throw out of the body. It is found that the skin throws off five out of eight pounds of the food and drink, or probably about three or four pounds a day. The lungs throw off one quarter as much as the skin, or about a pound a day. The remainder is carried off by the kidneys and lower intestines.

There is such a sympathy and connection between all the organs of the body, that when one of them is unable to work, the others perform the office of the feeble one. Thus, if the skin has its perspiration tubes closed up, then all the poisonous matter that would have been thrown out through them, must be emptied out either by the lungs, kidneys, or bowels.

When all these organs are strong and healthy, they can bear this increased labor without injury. But if the lungs are weak, the blood sent from the skin by the chill engorges the weak blood-vessels, and produces an inflammation of the lungs. Or it increases the discharge of a slimy mucous substance, that exudes from the skin of the lungs. This fills up the air-vessels, and would very soon end life, were it not for the spasms of the lungs, called *coughing*, which throws off this substance.

If, on the other hand, the bowels are weak, the chill on the skin, sending the blood into all the blood-vessels of the intestines, produces inflammation there, or else an excessive secretion of the mucous substance, which is called a *diarrhea*. Or if the kidneys are weak, there is an increased secretion and discharge from them, to an unhealthy and injurious extent.

This connection between the skin and internal organs is shown, not only by the effects of a chill on the skin, but by the sympathetic effect on itself when these internal organs suffer. For example, there are some kinds of food that will irritate and influence the stomach or the bowels, and this, by sympathy, will produce an immediate eruption on the skin.

Some persons, on eating strawberries, will immediately be affected with a nettle-rash. Others can not eat certain shell-fish without being affected in this way. Many humors on the face are caused by a diseased state of the internal organs with which the skin sympathizes.

This short account of the construction of the skin, and of its intimate connection with the internal organs, shows the philosophy of those modes of medical treatment that are addressed to this portion of the body.

It is on this powerful agency that the steam doctors rely, when, by moisture and heat, they stimulate all the innumerable perspiration tubes and lymphatics, to force out from the body a flood of unnaturally excited secretions; while it is "kill or cure," just as the chance may meet or oppose the demands of the case.

It is the skin also that is the chief basis of medical treatment in the Water Cure, whose slow processes are as much safer as they are slower.

At the same time it is the ill-treatment or neglect of the skin which, probably, are the causes of disease and decay to an incredible extent. The various particulars in which this may be seen, will be pointed out in the following pages.

LETTER NINTH.

It has been stated that the lungs and skin are the organs which provide and regulate the warmth of the body. The method by which this is done will now be explained.

There is an invisible agent called *caloric* or *heat*, which is the cause of warmth to the body, and every thing else. *Cola* is simply the want of this heat.

Caloric tends to diffuse itself equally; that is, whenever bodies have different degrees of heat, the caloric is constantly passing from the warmer to the colder substances, till they all come to the same temperature.

Thus, when we go into air colder than our bodies, the caloric passes from us to the surrounding atmosphere. But when we are surrounded by air, or touch any substance that is warmer than our bodies, the caloric passes from it to us. Clothes serve to prevent the heat from passing from our bodies to the air.

When water changes to ice, it gives out the caloric that kept it in a fluid state; and when it melts, and changes back to water, it takes the caloric required from the air or from objects that are around. This is the reason why it is so chilly often in a thaw. The caloric needed to melt the ice and snow is taken not only from the sun's rays, but from the air around.

When water changes to vapor, it takes in some caloric; and when vapor changes back to water, it gives out the caloric that held it in the vapor form. This, then, is the general rule in regard to changes made by caloric.

When a more solid body changes to a thinner or less dense one, caloric is absorbed; but when it changes from a less dense to a more solid form, caloric is given out.

There are certain changes that are made in combining

one body with another that produce heat.   Thus when cold water is poured into *aqua fortis*, or *sulphuric acid*, heat is produced by the mixture.

When oxygen combines with combustible bodies, heat is produced, and sometimes light.   Thus, when a candle burns, the light and heat are produced by the union of the oxygen of the air with the carbon of the tallow.   So, when wood or coal are burned, the light and heat are made by the union of the oxygen of the air with the carbon of the wood and coal.   .When we blow a fire it burns faster, because more air is thus furnished, from which the oxygen is taken.

The burning of any substance is its union with oxygen, and those bodies that can be thus burned are called combustibles.   Our bodies are composed chiefly of carbon, hydrogen, and nitrogen, which are combustibles, and also of oxygen, which unites with the other three.   This union always produces heat.

The blood, before it passes through the lungs, receives a supply of chyle from the stomach, and in the lungs it takes its supply of oxygen.   Then it passes to the capillaries, and there the oxygen unites with the decayed portions of the body, thus changing them to carbonic acid and water.   This is a process of combustion the same as when oxygen unites with wood or coal.   The oxygen of the new blood *burns* up a portion of the carbon and hydrogen in the capillaries, and *heat is given out*.   At the same time the fresh chyle is deposited in the place of the particles that are consumed.

The carbonic acid, formed by the combustion in the capillaries, and thrown out of the lungs and skin, is similar to the *smoke* of burning wood.   Another product of this combustion, which is drawn off from the blood by the kidneys, is similar to *ashes*.   Thus our bodies are kept warm by myriads of little fires in the innumerable capillaries.

In this process of warming the body, the stomach provides the fuel to burn, the lungs provide the oxygen to consume it, and the arteries carry the fuel and fire to the capillaries, where the combustion takes place.   The veins then carry off the carbonic acid, which, like smoke from a chimney, pours out of our mouth and nose and through the skin, while the kidneys empty out the ashes.

By this process of combustion in the capillaries the body is always kept nearly at a uniform temperature, which is about 98° by the thermometer. This is as warm as is the air in some of the hottest summer weather.

The air is usually cooler than our bodies, and is thus drawing off the caloric constantly. Clothing is useful only as it prevents the passing off of heat faster than the capillaries can keep up the supply.

We will now attend to the method by which the body is kept sufficiently cool.

It has been shown that the skin is filled with little perspiration tubes which are constantly sending off carbonic acid and water from the blood. The carbonic acid passes into the air, but much of the water is retained on the skin. Here the warmth of the body changes it to a vapor. In this change it abstracts its caloric from the body, and thus cools it. Thus the more heat is made in the capillaries the more perspiration is exhaled; and this being turned to vapor cools the body as fast as the capillaries heat it.

It is owing to this cooling process by the changing of perspiration to a vapor, that persons can stay in ovens hot enough to cook potatoes without being burned. The heat generates perspiration; this turns to vapor, and thus the body is cooled by the evaporation.

Thus the combustion in the capillaries keeps the body warmer than the surrounding air when it is cold, while if the air becomes hotter than the body, the emission and evaporation of perspiration keep it sufficiently cool.

We have now completed a description of some of the most important organs of the human body. Surely no one can have contemplated them, even in this imperfect exhibition, without the frequent exclamation, "How fearfully and wonderfully made!" At the same time, the laws by which these curiously-arranged and nicely-adjusted instruments of pain or happiness are to be made to fulfill their benevolent design, become the more important subjects of inquiry. These will be considered in the next letters.

PART SECOND

LETTER TENTH.

LAWS OF HEALTH AND HAPPINESS.

WE have attended to the construction of those organs of the body which are most important to health and happiness. We are now prepared to understand more readily the proper modes of using these organs in order to secure the highest degree of physical health and the happiness connected with it.

We call the rules for the proper use of these organs *the laws of health and happiness*, because our Creator has connected the reward of enjoyment with obedience to these rules, and the penalty of suffering with disobedience to them.

LAWS OF HEALTH FOR THE BONES.

It has been shown that the size, strength, and health of the bones, as well as every other part of the body, depend on good blood and pure air. If the stomach is supplied with unhealthy food, or if it is loaded with more than the body requires, the blood becomes impure, and consequently the bones, in common with all other parts, suffer more or less from this cause. So also if the air we breathe is loaded with the effluvia from the lungs and skin, or is diluted by excess of heat, the bones suffer with the rest of the system for want of oxygen and of properly prepared nutriment for the capillaries.

This shows the necessity of the following law of health for the bones : *Take care that the stomach has food of a proper kind and quality, and that the lungs are fully supplied with cool and pure air.*

We have learned that the bones also are in a measure

dependent on exercise for size and strength. A child that grows up with but little exercise will have bones that are softer and weaker than those of one who is trained to vigorous exercise. This debility will more readily induce deformity or disease from causes that would not affect a vigorous system. From this results the next law of health for the bones:

Take care that the body has sufficient exercise in pure air every day.

We have seen how curiously the spine is arranged with its vertebræ one above another, with the cartilage discs between, and the spinal marrow passing through the whole. Now it is indispensable to the health and perfect growth of the spine that it should have a great variety of motions, and that it never should be *habitually* kept out of its natural position. For any long-protracted unnatural position will frequently result in the hardening of the cartilage discs in the portions where they are thus compressed, until permanent distortion is induced. This shows the reason for the next law of health for the bones:

Take care that the spine shall never habitually be kept out of its natural position either when awake or asleep.

It has been shown, when the body is compressed around the waist, that the left side being over the stomach yields more readily than the right side, which is more firmly sustained by the liver. In consequence of this, the ribs of the left side are forced by any compression more strongly toward one side of the spine than toward the other. This makes a slow and steady *sidewise* pressure until the spine yields and the discs gradually harden, and a permanent *curvature of the spine* is the result. This is seen by the elevation of one shoulder and the projection of one hip.

Another result of tight dressing is the entire change in the shape of the thorax. The bones of the body in early life are soft and yielding. Constant pressure on the short ribs bring them nearer together in front, while the internal organs are pressed downward, reduced in size, and oftentimes misplaced.

This deformity of the thorax in a mother is often transmitted to her offspring as a hereditary misfortune, to be perpetuated from generation to generation.   This illustrates the importance of the next law of health for the bones:

Take care that the spine and thorax are not pressed into deformity by tight clothing around the waist.

LAWS OF HEALTH FOR THE MUSCLES.

It has been shown that the muscles, as well as every other part of the body, are nourished by the blood.   Consequently the health and strength of the muscles depend on the quality of the blood.   If the stomach is supplied with unhealthy food, or is loaded with more than is needed, unhealthy blood is the result.   And if the lungs are supplied with impure air, the capillaries in all parts of the body lose their life-giving oxygen, which alone can purify the body from its unhealthful portions.   Therefore the first law of health for the muscles is the same as for the bones:

Take care that the stomach has food of proper quality and quantity, and that the lungs are supplied with pure air.

We have seen that every movement of every muscle is attended with the decay of some of its particles, which must then be first changed by the oxygen brought by the arterial blood and then thrown out of the body through the lungs and skin. At the same time the fresh chyle takes the place of the particles thus removed.   It has also been shown that whenever a muscle is exercised the arterial blood flows more abundantly into it in order to furnish an increased supply of oxygen and chyle.   In this way the more the muscles are exercised the more strength and nourishment they receive from the blood, while they attain their full and perfect size.   This is the reason for the next law of health: *Take care that all the muscles of the body are brought to their full size and strength by a proper amount of exercise for each.*

The exercise of the muscles may be so prolonged that the decay of their particles will exceed the supply of nutrition furnished by the blood.   In this case the muscles will grow smaller and weaker from over-action.   Some persons injure themselves as much by excess of exercise as others do by the want of it.   This shows the reason for the next rule: *Take care that none of the muscles are weakened by excess of exercise.*

When the muscles have become small and feeble from want of proper exercise, a change in this respect must never be a sudden one. It should commence with but a small increase of exercise, and the daily additions should be very moderate. If this is not attended to, the muscles will be injured rather than benefited by increase of exercise. This is the reason for the next rule : *When an inactive habit of the muscular system is to be changed, it should be by a slow and gradual process.*

As increase of exercise increases the flow of blood to the muscles, it is very important that it should be done in pure and cool air. For if there is an increased amount of blood, and this blood has not been properly supplied with oxygen in the lungs, the action in the capillaries of the muscles is imperfect. This shows the importance of the next rule : *Never increase the ordinary amount of exercise till cool ana pure air is abundantly provided for the lungs.*

Light is very favorable to the perfect development of the human body. Vegetables that grow in the dark become pale and spindling; and so do children when they grow up in dark rooms and alleys of a city. This shows the reason for the next rule : *Let all vigorous exercise be taken by day light and not in the night.*

There is nothing more important to the health of certain muscles than a proper attitude in sitting and standing. In the natural position of the spine it is held in its upright form by its cartilage discs, so that there is no strain on any of the muscles of the trunk. But when we sit or stand crooked certain muscles are constantly in exercise to sustain the body in that position. After a habit of this kind is formed, the discs between the vertebræ gradually harden, and thus assist the muscles in their labor. But the result is, the spine becomes fixed in a deformed position, so that it can not be restored except by a long and laborious process.

But before this hardening process of the spine takes place the muscles that aid in supporting the spine are gradually reduced in strength, by constant labor in holding the body in an unnatural position. This shows the importance of the next rule : *Take care that the muscles of the trunk are not weakened by means of long-continued unnatural positions of the spine.*

Wherever any portion of the body is compressed by tight clothing the blood can not run freely into the muscles of that part. The consequence is, these muscles are reduced in size and strength. The muscles that sustain the spine should especially be protected from any such pressure. This shows the folly of attempting to cure crookedness or round shoulders by corsets or bracers. Any thing that compresses the muscles weakens them. The grand remedy for any such deformities, is *a proper training of the muscles in pure air.* Tight articles of dress around the neck, or legs, or arms, interfere with the full health and strength of the muscles. This shows the reason of the next rule : *Take care that the muscles, especially those of the trunk, be not weakened by any kind of tight dress.*

In cases where the muscles are injured, or are so weak that little exercise can be taken, rubbing, beating, and pinching them, so as to increase the flow of blood into them, is very important. There is nothing that so comforts and strengthens the weak as having the muscles rubbed and otherwise exercised by intermitting pressure, especially when it can be done in pure air and after a bath.

In hot countries, where the inhabitants are too indolent to use their own muscles in the proper way, it is deemed a great luxury to take a bath and then have the muscles kneaded, pinched, and otherwise manipulated by bath attendants. This shows the reason for the next rule : *When a person is too weak to use the muscles, let another person increase the flow of blood into them by manipulations.*

There is nothing so indispensable to beauty of form as the *proper* exercise of *all* the muscles. It is rarely, if ever, the case in this nation that any care is taken in this respect. Children, in their sports, do not fail—especially if they have full run in the country—to accomplish this; but grown persons generally confine their exercise to a small portion of the body. In this way the perfect and rounded form of childhood is rarely preserved to mature life as it might be with proper care. This shows the need of the next rule : *Let special care be directed to the universal development of all the muscles during the period of childhood and youth, and take care that, all through life, the muscles of the whole body be duly exercised.*

LETTER ELEVENTH.

WE have seen that the lungs have two offices to perform: one is, to prepare the food sent from the stomach by adding the oxygen of the air to the chyle; the other is, the emptying out from the body the carbonic acid and water which is formed in the capillaries by the union of this oxygen with the decayed particles of the body. The combination of oxygen with carbon and hydrogen in the capillaries also produces the animal heat which keeps the body warmer than the air around us.

Every inspiration takes in about half a pint of fresh air, which is added to the air already in the lungs, this being about three pints. We inspire about twenty times every minute, taking about one hogshead of new air into the lungs every hour, and expire the same quantity of bad air. Thus every pair of lungs requires, every hour, a hogshead of pure air, and vitiates the same quantity.

Carbonic acid is a little heavier than common air; but when it is mixed and warmed, as it is in our lungs, it becomes lighter than the surrounding cooler atmosphere and rises. Thus, in large assemblies in churches, the air at the upper part of the room is more impure than that below, which is supplied with air from without by the doors and windows. When cold and warm air are brought together, the warm air rises and the cold air presses downward. This is the cause of the motion in air which keeps the carbonic acid from accumulating in any one place where many people are breathing.

But the more the air is warmed, and the more houses are made close so that the outer air can not enter, the more the breathing of those in these houses increases the carbonic acid and uses up the oxygen.

As has been said, every pair of lungs vitiates a hogshead of air every hour; and therefore this quantity of pure air is needed each hour, by every individual, both by night and by day, in order to secure the most perfect health and enjoyment of life.

There is no way in which houses can be supplied with pure air but by some mode of ventilation which secures the continuous entrance and exit of as much pure air as is breathed by the inmates of these houses. Of course, the more persons are in one room or one house, the greater necessity of increased ventilation.

The introduction of warm air at the bottom of a room, and the construction of properly-placed ventilators for the escape of this air out of the room, is a sure mode of supplying a room with pure air. But unless great care is taken, the air thus heated will be too dry and too warm.

Open fire-places, that make a constant draught of the air of a room upward and outward, insure a constant supply of fresh air from the doors and windows.

But close stoves, with tight doors and windows, make it almost certain that the inmates of a room will constantly breathe impure air, which will act as a slow poison in undermining the constitution. And when the constitution is thus weakened diseases of all sorts find ready entrance.

These remarks illustrate this law of health for the lungs: *Every pair of lungs should have a supply of pure air at the rate of one hogshead for every hour.*

It has been shown that there are two processes for filling the lungs: one by the expanding outward and upward of the ribs; and the other by the action of the diaphragm and the muscles of the abdomen. Of course, any tight clothing around the ribs prevents their action in breathing; and tight dressing around the lower part of the body serves also to lessen the abdominal breathing. All such compressions make it certain that a portion of the air-cells of the lungs will never receive any air. In consequence of this the blood will not be properly supplied with oxygen, and the constitution is gradually weakened. This illustrates the importance of the next law of health : *The body should never be so constrained by the dress as to impede, in the least degree, the movement of the ribs or abdominal muscles in breathing.*

It has been shown how the body may be so altered in form as to become permanently crooked, and the shoulders rounded. Both these distortions diminish the space allowed to the lungs. A person with bent back must have the lungs, stomach, and abdomen pressed together in front so as to diminish the capacity for a full inflation ; while round shoulders make a flat and narrow chest, and give little space for the lungs. This shows the importance of the next law of health for the lungs : *The habitual positions of the body in walking, sitting, and sleeping should be such as to give full expansion to the lungs in breathing.*

It is probable that there is no law of health so universally violated by all classes of persons as the one which demands that every pair of lungs should have fresh air at the rate of a hogshead an hour. If all the poisonous matter that pours from nose and mouth, and exhales from the skin, were *colored*, so as to be visible, and we should see a black or blue vapor accumulating around us as fast as the air of a room was vitiated, there would be an instant change in the feeling and conduct of mankind.

But as it is, the decayed particles of our bodies are floating about us, and accumulating around our sleeping pillows, every day and every night. At every inspiration we take in air thus adulterated, which is spread through the multitudinous air-cells, whose membraneous extent equals the floor of a room twelve feet square, and then is expired with a still larger amount of unhealthful mixture.

And the richer our people grow the tighter they make their doors and windows, and the more they multiply stoves in sitting and sleeping rooms, and the less they exercise in pure air. While in some wretched country hovel the poor drink abundantly the life-inspiring and pure breath of heaven every hour of the day and night, the children of wealth sip it only for.an hour or two, as they ride abroad in their luxurious equipages for " exercise and air."

LETTER TWELFTH.

WE have seen that the nourishment for the body is prepared in the stomach and other intestines, and then carried through the lacteals and thoracic duct to a large vein which conducts it to the heart. Then it passes from the heart to the lungs, to obtain oxygen from the veins, which completes its preparation.

The health of the body is greatly dependent on the *kina* of food taken, some being much more favorable to health than others; and we will first notice some facts that are useful to guide in the proper selection of nourishment.

ANIMAL AND VEGETABLE FOOD.

All kinds of food are composed chiefly of the four elements, *oxygen*, *hydrogen*, *carbon*, and *nitrogen*. It is the *different proportions* in which these elements are combined that cause all the varieties which exist in both animal and vegetable food. Wheat and potatoes, for example, have precisely the same ingredients as beef or any other meat, only in different proportions.

But the health of the body requires that, in certain circumstances, one kind of food, in which one of these elements abounds shall be avoided, while in other cases it is necessary.

HEAT-FORMING AND FLESH-FORMING FOOD.

The two purposes of food are, first, to supply the nourishment that takes the place of the old and decayed particles of the body; and, second, to furnish the fuel needed in the capillaries to warm the body. When the atmosphere is warm, less heat needs to be manufactured within; but in very cold air a large supply of carbon and oxygen must be carried to the capillaries, to supply the heat that is carried off by the surrounding atmosphere. With reference to this, food is divided into the two classes called *heat-forming* and *flesh-forming*. Those substances that contain the most *carbon* are those which best supply fuel for warming the body. Among these, sugar, molasses, the fat of animals, butter, and oils of all kinds, are the most common. On the other hand, the flesh of animals divested of the fat, and some of the vegetables, have least carbon.

From this it is manifest that it is needful to regulate the food with reference to the quantity of carbon required to warm the body. If an excess is taken into the system, all the organs are overworked in throwing it off.

Nitrogen is one of the ingredients of muscle or flesh, and therefore no animal can live a long time on food which is destitute of this element.

The flesh of animals furnishes this element in larger proportion than vegetable food. But nitrogen is a constituent in wheat, rye, oats, potatoes, and various vegetables, though not in so large a proportion as in animal food. Thus animal and vegetable food both supply all the elements needed for the perfect health of the body, and we need only proper knowledge and self-control to regulate the selection according as circumstances vary.

STIMULATING FOOD.

It is found that those articles which contain the most nitrogen have a quality which is called *stimulating*. Such food makes the heart beat quicker, and all the organs of the body work faster than less stimulating articles. The most stimulating of all food is the flesh of animals, which, as before stated, contains more nitrogen than any other article.

NOURISHING FOOD.

Articles that contain, in a given weight, the largest amount of the elements that both warm and nourish the body, are the most nourishing or nutritious. There are calculations made by chemists which show the amount of nourishment in each article of food. By these it appears that the common idea that animal food contains more nourishment than vegetable is incorrect.

E

Beans and peas are found to have more nutriment in a given weight than any other common food. And wheat and rye flour have more nourishment in a given weight than beef, or any kind of meat. It is the *stimulating* property of meat which has led to the impression that it is more nourishing than a vegetable diet.

The tables made by chemists, giving the amount of nutriment in each kind of food, show that while the flesh of animals (not the fat) in every hundred pounds has twenty-five of solid matter to seventy-five of water, bread has just the reverse; that is, seventy-five pounds of solid matter to twenty-five pounds of water.

All the experiments that have been made show also that vegetable food digests quicker than animal. Thus, in the case of St. Martin, bean soup, boiled rice, potatoes, stale bread, and several other articles, digested sooner than any kind of meat or any kind of meat broth.

The working people in almost every nation are obliged to live almost entirely on vegetable diet, because it is so much cheaper; for it takes fifteen times as much land to provide animal food as it does to supply a vegetable diet. The working people in Ireland live on potatoes. The peasantry of Lancashire and Cheshire, who are the handsomest race in England, live chiefly on potatoes and butter-milk. The bright and hardy Arabs live almost entirely on vegetable food. The brave and vigorous Spartans never ate meat. Most of the hardiest soldiers in Northern Europe seldom taste of meat. From the creation to this day more than two-thirds of mankind never have eaten animal food; and, except in America, it is rare that the strongest laborers eat any meat.

It is also a fact, that when, in past time, various great men wished to have their heads unusually clear for intellectual labor, they gave up animal food.

These things are stated, not to prove that animal food is not suitable, nor that, in some cases and for some purposes, it is not better than an exclusively vegetable diet, but to aid in removing the false notion that meat is *more nourishing* than other food, and to show that it is not necessary to the perfect development both of mind and body.

When men, from any cause, need to be not only nourished but *stimulated* by food, then animal food is the best. When they need to have their body well nourished, and yet not stimulated, then vegetable food is the best.

HIGHLY CONCENTRATED FOOD AND INNUTRITIOUS FOOD.

There is a certain amount of *bulk* necessary to enable the stomach to perform the digestive process. For this reason, food that is so highly concentrated as to supply much nutrition in little space is not healthful. In order to render such articles digestible there must be a certain mixture of innutritious matter, that passes through the intestines without digestion or assimilation. The use of such innutritious food is to increase the bulk and to stimulate the organs. It is owing to this that bread of unbolted wheat is more easily digested than that made of fine wheat.

DIGESTIBLE FOOD.

Food is digestible in proportion to the facility with which it is acted on by the gastric juice.

Some articles of food that contain abundant nourishment really yield but a small supply, because they do not easily digest; while others, that digest more readily, afford more nourishment, though their relative amount of nutriment is small. It is owing to this fact that those kinds of meat which digest readily are more nourishing, in certain states of the stomach, than much more nutritive articles, such as beans and peas, which are more difficult of digestion.

The above facts in regard to the nature of different kinds of food, are the foundation of the rules that are to guide in its selection.

RULES FOR SELECTING FOOD.

If any person is confined exclusively to one kind of food, it should be one which combines all the elements required in nourishing all parts of the body. Experiments have been tried on dogs and cats, which show that an animal fed exclusively on fat, or sugar, or any article that is chiefly carbon, without any nitrogen, will become unhealthy, and live but a short time.

Milk and eggs have all the elements needed by the body in good proportions. So have wheat, rye, corn, potatoes, and many other vegetables, as well as some of the fruits. This rule, then, is important : *There should always be such variety in food as to furnish all the elements needed to nourish the body.*

In a warm climate the body does not need much heat generated within. And the air, being diluted with heat, contains less oxygen to burn the carbon in the capillaries. In reference to this, food that contains much carbon, such as oil, sugar, fat, and the like, should be avoided. And as heat is stimulating and exhausting, it is important that the food taken in warm weather should be cooling and unstimulating. For this reason, in a hot season or climate, animal food, which is the most stimulating of any, should be avoided, and the diet consist chiefly of bread, fruits, and vegetables, which are nourishing but not stimulating. As cold weather comes on, meat and oily substances may be eaten with more safety. Then, again, when spring returns, they should be relinquished, or reduced in quantity. This rule, then, is important : *The selection of food should vary with temperature and seasons.*

The organs of young children are more sensitive and excitable than those of mature persons. For this reason, a nutritious diet of milk, bread, fruit, and vegetables is more suitable than stimulating animal food.

Regard should also be paid to *temperament*, both in children and in adults. Some persons are of a very excitable temperament, and such insure longer life and better health by a nourishing, unstimulating diet. Others are cool, slow, and phlegmatic. Such can safely eat more stimulating food, and, in certain cases, it is more healthful than any other. A person of full habit and excitable temperament, in order to secure long life, should be confined almost exclusively to a diet of bread, fruit, and vegetables. This rule, then, is important : *In selecting food regard should be had to age and temperament.*

The state of health, especially of the digestive organs, is to be regarded. When there is a tendency to constipation, highly concentrated food, such as candies, cakes, rice, and fine flour, should be avoided, and fruits, coarse bread, and vegetables be sought. When there is a tendency to diarrhea, then rice, fine flour, and other concentrated food should be sought, and fruits and vegetables avoided.

When the digestive organs are very sensitive and easily affected, it is important to adopt an unstimulating, yet nutritious diet as soon as warm weather approaches. Many young children would be saved from early death by attention to these rules. Owing to habit or constitution some kinds of food are better adapted to the stomach of one person than to that of others. Experience is a better guide than theories. Such food as disturbs the stomach should be avoided, whatever it may be. And food that is difficult to digest should be wholly avoided, especially by those of delicate constitution or poor health, for nothing taxes all the organs of the body so much as food that will not digest properly, and yet must in some way be carried out of the body.

Universal experience has shown that unmixed and simple food digests more easily than rich and complicated articles. New bread is far more difficult of digestion than stale, because mastication changes it to a compact dough form, which does not readily unite with the gastric juice. It is quite the reverse with stale bread. Oils and fats are much more difficult to digest when cooked than in their natural state. All articles made rich with butter, sugar, and spices, are difficult to digest. From these facts the following rule is derived: *In selecting food regard should be had to its relative digestibility and to the state of health, especially of the digestive organs.*

ON THE QUANTITY OF FOOD.

Physicians and physiologists maintain that there is more sickness and death caused by excess in the *quantity* of food taken than by the violation of any other law of health. The reason of this is that men have so abused nature that *appetite* has ceased to be a guide to most persons as to the amount of food needed. Mankind collect a great variety of articles to tempt the palate, and then eat one thing after another till they feel full, and can eat no more. In this way the stomach receives far more than is required to nourish the body, and thus the nervous powers, together with the lungs, kidneys, bowels, skin, and lymphatics, are over-taxed to throw out of the system this excess. The energies of the body are slowly and gradually worn down by this excess of useless labor.

The following presents the rules to guide in reference to the *quantity* of food:

Persons who labor or exercise any way demand more food than those of sedentary habits. Whenever, therefore, any changes are made from active to sedentary habits, great care should be taken to diminish the quantity of food. This is especially important to young persons, who change from active home-duties to the inactive habits of students. Such ought to deny themselves, even when their appetite would lead to as large an allowance as common. Thus, in a short time, the appetite will accommodate to the real wants of the body. The fact that the stomach of most persons in this nation of plenty has been so accustomed to more food than the system requires, is the reason why the appetite can not guide, and reason must take its place. Most persons eat more than they need, and the stomach accommodates till a habit is formed. And then there may be a feeling of *emptiness*, even when food is not needed.

The great preservative against excess in food is a *simple diet*. When the food is plain, and no tempting variety stimulates the palate, most persons will take only what the wants of the system require. But where there is a succession of articles, and those of a tempting nature, almost every person will eat more than is needful, and thus overtask the organs of the body in throwing off the excess.

There is a class of articles called *condiments*, that stimulate the appetite to an unnatural degree. Pepper, mustard, and spices, are those most commonly used. These articles have very little nourishment, are entirely needless, and always tend to create a false appetite. Besides this, they are inflammatory in their nature, and stimulating to the nervous system. The excessive use of salt, sugar, and molasses, is a method of stimulating the appetite by food which, in proper quantities, is healthful. Articles preserved in salt, sugar, or vinegar, are neither as easily digested, nor as healthful as those in the natural state. In reference to these facts, the following rule is very important: *The quantity of food should vary with the amount of exercise taken, and excess should be guarded against by a simple diet, and the avoidance of condiments.*

ON THE TIME AND MANNER OF TAKING FOOD.

There is no way in which children have their stomachs weakened so frequently as by irregular and frequent eating. None of the muscles of the body are taxed so severely as those of the stomach, and they need periods of rest. If, therefore, there is a constant entrance of food into the stomach, there is no time for rest, while there is a constant mixture of partly-digested and newly-arrived food that interrupts the natural process of digestion. From two to three hours pass before the stomach ceases its muscular action, and then it needs two or three hours to rest. The meals, therefore, should be five or six hours apart for grown persons. Children, who are growing, and whose organs act faster, may eat a small luncheon between meals with advantage, if they feel hungry enough to eat bread alone, but not otherwise. The above shows the importance of the following rule : *Food should be taken at regular times, and at intervals of five or six hours. No food should be put into the stomach while the digestive process is incomplete.*

It has been shown that whenever any of the muscles are exercised, the blood flows more abundantly to them to supply the nourishment needed. Every movement of a muscle hastens the decay of its particles, and increases the demand for fresh nutriment. Therefore, when the stomach has a full meal to digest, a portion of the blood must leave other parts of the body for this service. But if during the time of digestion the muscles of the body are thrown into vigorous exercise, they draw off the blood, and thus the stomach is robbed of its proper proportion. So if the brain is set to work vigorously after a full meal, it draws off the blood which is needed by the stomach. This shows the need of the following rule : *Immediately after eating a full meal, vigorous exercise, either of body or mind, should be avoided.* Slight exercise, like riding, or agreeable mental activity, such as lively conversation, are favorable to good digestion.

When the body is exhausted by labor or vigorous exercise, the stomach should not be called upon to commence the labor of digestion. For the nervous energies of the whole system have been employed in labor, and there is not a proper supply for the stomach till a period of rest intervenes. So after protracted mental labor, the whole body needs a period of repose before the stomach can properly be called to labor. This shows the reason for the following rule: *A half hour or an hour of rest should intervene after vigorous exercise, either of mind or body, before eating.*

During the period of sleep, the brain being inactive does not send out its supply of nervous fluid as in waking hours, and consequently all the functions of life go on slower, and the system has not its full power. This is shown by the respiration, which is slower during sleep than at other times. Of course the stomach shares in this temporary diminution of power. Though many persons have strong stomachs, so that they can digest food well even in the feebler hours of sleep, still it is imposing labor on the stomach at a wrong time. This is especially injurious to such as have a weak constitution or weak digestive powers. The following rule then is important: *Let two or three hours intervene between eating and sleeping.*

The position of the body has an important influence on the health of the stomach. A habit of standing and sitting crooked interferes with the functions of the stomach and bowels. These organs are thus crowded into an unnatural position, and have not room to perform their operations properly. Therefore the following rule is important: *Be careful not to interfere with the process of digestion by bad positions of the body.*

There is no portion of the body so intimately connected with the stomach and the liver as *the skin.* We have shown that the lining of the stomach and intestines is in fact only a continuation of the outer skin. The custom of physicians to examine the tongue results from the fact of a sympathy which exists between the interior skin and the skin of the tongue, so that any diseased state within the body extends more or less to the mouth, especially to the tongue. This sympathy between the outer and inner skin makes it important to the stomach that we should, by ablution and all other methods, keep the outer skin in perfect health. Therefore the following rule is important: *Attend to the health ana purity of the skin as one mode of securing a healthy stomach.*

It has been shown that the process of respiration, when perfect and natural, involves the mutual action of the diaphragm and abdominal muscles, by which the lower intestines are constantly kept in gentle motion. This is a very important stimulus to the process of digestion. Of course any mode of dress that restrains the movement of the ribs and abdominal muscles interferes with this process. From this results the importance of this rule: *Be careful not to interrupt the process of digestion by tight clothing around the middle or lower portions of the body.*

The health and well-being of all the organs of digestion and nutrition very much depend upon the *daily* evacuation of the lower intestines. *Regular habits* in this respect should be formed and carefully preserved. Such arrangements should be made in every family and in every school, that no person shall ever be obliged to delay when nature prompts to this necessary duty. Such delays always tend to produce constipation. Every parent and every teacher should carefully guard the young from such violations of the laws of health. There is no rule of health more important than this: *Take all proper methods to prevent constipation.*

The experiments in the Water Cure establishments prove that some notions in regard to drink have been mistaken ones. It has been shown that veins of the stomach draw off the superfluous liquids before digestion commences. A pint of water will be thus taken off in five or six minutes, as has been witnessed in experiments made on St. Martin, a man who had a large opening made into his stomach, which healed up in such a way that all the processes within could be seen.

When liquid food—such as broths, soups, or juicy fruits—are taken, the first process is the absorption of the excess of liquid. This shows that no special harm is done by taking drink with our meals. It is as well to eat solid food and drink water at the same time, as to take bread and milk or eat soup and broth. In either case, the stomach performs the same duty, and removes the excess of liquid. Very cold drinks interrupt the digestive process, and should not be taken while eating.

The notion, too, that there is any danger from drinking freely of *cold* water at times when the stomach is empty, is also exploded by multitudes of experiments. Nothing is more serviceable to digestion, or better promotes the healthful action of all the functions of the body, than drinking two or three tumblers of cold water before a meal, especially before breakfast. There is no danger of "thinning the blood" so long as the kidneys perform their office of removing from the body any excess of liquids. Pure cold water is a tonic to the capillaries, and instead of thinning, tends to purify the blood. It is also a remedy for constipation and inaction of the liver.

The rules, therefore, that have been given by some writers and physicians, not to drink freely of cold water, are not founded on a correct philosophy or a sufficiently extended observation.

There is no way in which the stomach and whole body has been so much abused as by the use of stimulating drinks. It is found by the experience of ages, that alcohol and opium, tea and coffee, simply stimulate the brain and nervous system, and furnish little or no nourishment. This stimulus is always followed by a reaction of debility, which is proportioned to the degree of previous stimulation.

The body always accommodates, more or less, to any kind of abuse, so that such stimulants may be taken often and long without any immediate or perceptible injury. But this no more justifies the use of these articles than it does the taking of arsenic or any other poison to which the body may in some degree become habituated. In some countries of Europe the people use small quantities of arsenic, because the first effect is both to stimulate and to increase flesh and beauty of countenance. And when the habit and a love of the excitement are thus formed, the practice is continued, though emaciation and death are the final results. Animals, having no reason to guide them, are formed so that they usually have an instinct to warn them from those kinds of food that would harm them. But man, having reason bestowed for his guidance, is expected to form habits of virtue and self-control, so that when experience shows any practice to be pernicious it will be avoided.

There is nothing so abundantly proved as that narcotic and alcoholic drinks are never needed except as medicinal agents, and that their habitual use always tends to injury and excess. Men are debilitated by alcoholic drinks and tobacco. Women are almost as much injured in their health and comfort by the use of tea and coffee. Multitudes of wives and mothers become feeble, irritable, and miserable from the daily exhaustion caused by these narcotic stimulants. They feel the loss of their tea or coffee almost as much as the inebriate misses his daily libations. And yet they are so ignorant of physiology as often to imagine that the little strength they have is the gift of the baneful cups which yield only poison. They drink and feel better because a new stimulus is applied to the brain and nerves, to be followed by a new, secret, but certain drain on their nervous fountain. This law of health, then, is imperious: *Never use stimulating drinks except for medicinal purposes.*

LETTER THIRTEENTH.

LAWS OF HEALTH. THE SKIN AND SECRETING ORGANS.

WE have attended to the curious and wonderful construction of the skin, and the various important functions it fulfills in protecting the body, in acting as the organ of touch, in purifying the blood, and in warming or cooling the body as its varying temperature may require.

Inasmuch as so large an amount of unhealthful matter is to be sent out of the system through the skin, we can perceive the importance of keeping the pores, which are its outlets, free from all accumulations. The pressure of the clothing tends to confine these excretions to the surface, while heat and warmth stimulate the lymphatics to absorb any thing on the skin. Thus a double evil may ensue, in preventing the outflow of unhealthful matter, and the reabsorbing of what is already sent out. This shows the importance of this rule: *Take care that every portion of the skin is purified by washing the whole body at least once a day.*

It has been stated that there is more blood in the capillaries of the skin than in those of all the rest of the body. This being the case, there is nothing more accessory to the equalization and proper circulation of the blood, than that the capillaries of the skin be at all times well filled. Nothing is a surer sign of perfect health than a skin whose capillaries are in full circulation. And whenever any internal trouble exists, the main reliance for relief should be to draw the blood to the skin, and thus reduce the internal inflammation. All inflammations are the effect of the engorgement of the capillaries with an excess of blood.

This shows the philosophy of the steam-doctor's cure, in certain cases, and of the use of blisters. The steaming of the whole body brings the blood into the skin, and thus inflamed internal organs are relieved, and much bad matter thrown off through the pores. Blisters are put on the skin near the place where some internal inflammation exists, and by exciting another point excessively, draw the blood from the inflamed part. Thus, inflammation on the lungs can sometimes be relieved by a blister on the chest. But both these remedies involve evils, and are inferior to certain *safe* processes of the Water Cure that will hereafter be explained.

This shows the reason for the next law of health : *Whenever.the body has been in any way chilled, and internal disorder results, relief should be sought by drawing the blood into the capillaries of the skin.*

It has been found that both *light* and *air* are healthful tonics to the skin. A child that grows up in a dark cellar or any dark room, will always have a pale and unhealthy countenance. The effect of air and light in strengthening the skin is shown by the face and exposed parts of the neck, which become so strong to bear changes of temperature as scarcely to feel them. This shows another advantage of universal washing of the person, as thus the skin obtains an *air bath,* and the genial influence of *light.* There is much advantage, also, in prolonging the exposure of the skin to the air, so long as it can be done, and yet retain a warm and healthful glow. But as soon as a chilly feeling commences, the clothing should be resumed. The object of clothing is to prevent the animal heat generated in the capillaries from passing to the surrounding air. If there is too little covering, then the skin becomes chilled, and its pores closed, and we *take a cold.* Sometimes, when one part of the body is chilled, the cold settles in some of the muscles whose capillaries are engorged by the blood retreating from the skin. This is called a *rheumatism.* Sometimes the capillaries of the nerve-cases become engorged by a chill, and this is one species of neuralgia. Sometimes the face has been chilled, and then the capillaries of the teeth and jaws become engorged, and toothache ensues. These particulars show the reasons for the following rule : *Take care to save all parts of the body from chills that will close the pores.*

It has been found by experience, that when cold water is applied to the skin, there is, in good health, an immediate contraction of the capillaries, which sends the blood for an instant inward · but immediately there is a reaction of the system, which returns the blood to the skin in greater quantities. This has the same benefit on the capillaries of the skin which exercise has on the muscles. It increases their capacity of holding blood, and their action in sending off bad material, and replacing it with new; and it is thus the skin of the face and neck are strengthened to bear changes of temperature without feeling uncomfortable or being injured.

On the contrary, it has been found by experience, that the application of heat to the skin, though it draws the blood into the capillaries, does it by a process that debilitates instead of strengthening. Thus, a person in good health may take a cold bath every day, and gain vigor. But if he should take a hot bath as often and as long, it would debilitate. It has been found, however, that if a hot bath is followed by a cold one, this debilitating influence on the skin is lessened. As a general rule, then, cold is a tonic to the skin, and heat debilitates it. From this follows the next rule of health for the skin : *Take care that no part of the body be kept so warm by clothing as to debilitate it by excess of heat.*

It has been found, also, that the power of the body to bear cold depends much upon habit. When the skin has been kept very warm with too much clothing, it becomes very sensitive to cold. On the contrary, cold bathing, and light clothing, and frequent exposures to the cold air, so strengthen the whole body, and especially the skin, that very much less clothing is needed than where the habits are the reverse. So persons who take a great deal of exercise outdoors, generate so much animal heat, and have their skin so strengthened by cold air, that they require much less clothing than those who go out but little, exercise but little, and keep their skins overheated by fires and clothing. This rule, then, is important : *Take care to keep the body warm by exercise, cool air, and bathing, instead of relying on clothing and fires, which tend to debilitate the skin.*

There is always danger of *excess* in applying the foregoing rules. Some constitutions are so weak that they have not nervous power enough to bear much exercise, or to resist the cold. Many such have been seriously injured by cold bathing, by exposures to cold weather, and by deficient clothing. There is almost an unerring index to guide such in these attempts to secure good habits in the above particulars. Whenever the skin is too delicate, or the body too feeble to bear cold bathing, there is a sensation of discomfort, a chilliness, or a consequent debility, which should immediately be heeded. And so in regard to clothing and exposure to the air. Whatever makes a person chilly and uncomfortable should be avoided. There should always be a slow and cautious method pursued in all attempts to change the habits, especially in the management of the skin.

A delicate person, unaccustomed to expose the skin to cold air and cold water, should begin to bathe in a warm room, and use tepid water at first, and follow bathing with a good deal of friction. Then each day the water should very slowly and gradually be reduced in temperature, and the air of the room in warmth. This rule, therefore, is very important: *Never use water so cold or clothing so thin as to cause a sense of chilliness and discomfort. Change the habits in these respects very slowly, and always stop when discomfort is induced.*

In regard to bathing, it must be remembered that, while warm bathing tends to debilitate, cold bathing draws off the animal heat, and may be carried to such an extent as to undermine the constitution. Many children have been seriously injured by bathing too often, or staying too long in cold water. The animal heat is thus drawn off faster than the powers of the body can supply it, and the process becomes debilitating. So, while some children have their skin weakened by wearing too much clothing, both while sleeping and waking, others are equally injured by being forced to go about chilly from want of enough covering. In general, young children need more clothing than adults. This is a safe rule: *Keep as little clothing on children as is consistent with their comfort, but add more when they complain of chilliness.*

Age and disease both reduce the powers of the system to generate heat and to react when cold is applied. For this reason *the invalid and the aged should wear more clothing than the young and vigorous, and be more cautious in using cola baths.*

Currents of air on certain parts of the body are more injurious than a general cooling of the whole body. The reason is, that heat is withdrawn much faster by a current of air than by a still atmosphere. And when this current is confined to a small portion of the body, it causes the blood to retreat from that to the inner organs, and thus renders the circulation unequal, and the system less prepared to act vigorously against the evil. This rule, therefore, is important: *Currents of air on the head or neck, or any particular part of the body should be avoided. Any part of the body that has been habitually covered, should not be exposed without a gradual process to inure it to the change. Any change in amount of clothing worn should be made in the morning, because the body is then most vigorous.*

It has become a very prevalent notion that it is dangerous to bathe or to go into the cold air when the skin is very warm. This has arisen from the fact that in a perspiration, the clothing being wet, cold air carries off the heat much faster than when the clothing is dry. At the same time, the sweating process sometimes proceeds so far as to debilitate the skin.

But the experience of Water Cures has proved that the best time to bathe is when the skin is warm and flushed with exercise.

It is when the capillaries are filled with blood that the nerves and blood-vessels are at their highest point of vigor. On the contrary, when the skin is cool there is less blood and less vigor to resist cold.

This rule, then, is important: *When the body is to be suddenly exposed to cold air or cold water, the capillaries of the skin should be filled with blood by exercise or friction.*

As the impurities of the body sent out through the skin collect in the clothing and bedding, and as the absorbents of the skin take back impurities that are pressed on to it, it is very important that the clothing should be changed often. And as fresh air has a direct effect in carrying off these impurities, it is important that bedding and clothing should be well aired. This rule, then, is necessary: *Take care to air the bedding and night-clothes, and to change frequently the garments worn next the skin.*

Inasmuch as there is more blood in the capillaries of the skin than in all t e other capillaries of the whole body, we can see how important it is to the health of this organ that the stomach should be supplied with proper food and in proper quantities. It is probable that most evils that are developed in cutaneous eruptions, result from excess in eating, or from a wrong selection of food. This rule, then, is important: *Take care that the health of the skin be secured by moderate supplies of properly selected food.*

It has been shown that the skin is intimately connected with the lungs, liver, kidneys, and bowels, and that any abuse of any one of these may affect the health of any of the others. Whenever, therefore, any internal organ suffers, care should immediately be taken that all the functions of the skin are in full and perfect operation. And special caution should be directed to prevent any increase of disease by any chill of the skin.

In climates that are deemed unhealthy, or where unhealthy miasmas abound, special care should be taken that the skin be kept clean, and the capillaries well-filled by exercise, food, and warmth. In moving among contagious disorders, the keeping of the skin clean and warm, and properly nourished by simple and wholesome food, is the surest preventive from disease. This rule, then, is important: *In times of sickness or of exposure to epidemic or contagious disease, take great care to keep the skin clean, and warm, and well-nourished.*

We have seen that the secreting tubes of the skin that draw off the unhealthful portions of the blood amount, if all united, to *twenty-eight miles* in length. All this apparatus is dependent on the purity of the air to secure the requisite amount of oxygen for the performance of its functions. There is no portion of the body that suffers more directly and severely from an impure atmosphere than the skin. This rule, then, is imperative: *Guard the health of the skin by at all times surrounding it with pure air.*

LAWS OF HEALTH. THE BRAIN AND NERVES.

We have seen that the brain and nerves are the organs by which the mind controls the other parts of the body. We have also seen that they are divided into distinct portions, each having different offices to perform, and that a

F

nervous fluid generated in the brain is the medium of influence between the mind, and brain, and nerves.

We have seen that the fountain that supplies this fluid may be so overdrawn by excesses as to be exhausted, and also that certain portions of the brain and nervous system may be overworked, and thus debilitated, while other portions may become equally debilitated by inaction.

Before proceeding to set forth the laws of health for the brain and nerves, some preliminary remarks are needful in reference to the nature of true happiness, and the mode of attaining it.

We will first assume, what probably few will dispute, that in the formation of our minds and bodies, our benevolent and wise Creator aimed to secure to his creatures the best happiness by the best methods, and that he has placed us in a system wisely adapted to secure this end. Being thus endowed and thus placed, we are to learn, by our own experience and that of others, how we are to use our various powers and susceptibilities so as to secure the happiness which we are formed to enjoy.

By this experience we have learned that there are two methods which may be adopted. One is to seek and enjoy, temperately, a great variety of intellectual, social, and moral pleasures, giving to each its due proportion, and allowing no injurious excess in any. Where this course is pursued the happiness of life is made up of multitudes of successive enjoyments, no one of which is very exciting or ecstatic, but the united sum producing a calm, steady, satisfying happiness.

By the other method all the feelings and energies are directed to a few objects, which, if secured, are enjoyed to excess, while other resources remain closed, and the mind is unharmoniously developed.

Experience also teaches that there are some kinds of happiness much more elevating and satisfying than others. Thus intellectual pleasures exceed those of a merely physical nature, social pleasures are superior to selfish, while moral and religious enjoyments are the most elevating and perfect of them all.

True and abiding happiness, then, is to be found in the proper and equal development and exercise of all the fac-

ulties of body and mind, and in the appropriate selection
and proportion of the objects of enjoyment.

We will now consider the laws of health for the brain
and nerves.

One of the most important of these laws is what has been
.repeated in reference to every other portion of the body.
The quality of the blood that nourishes the brain depends
on the right selection and quality of food, and on the full
supply of oxygen which pure air alone can afford.   When
the blood is surcharged with heavy and gross material from
excess in diet, it clogs the operations, and impedes the
health of the brain and nervous system.   And when the air
inspired by the lungs is impure, the brain loses in the same
proportion its healthful stimulus.   The brain never acts
so free and clear as in a perfectly pure atmosphere, while
dullness and debility are the certain results of impure air.
I have known a teacher, who, when he found his class in
mathematics weary and perplexed with a difficult problem,
instantly relieve them, and secure a speedy result, by letting
down the tops of the windows, and thus sending a fresh supply of oxygen to the brain.   Pure air adds as much to every
other enjoyment as it does to the exercise of the intellect.
This rule, then, may stand as first : *Take care that the brain
is nourished with healthful blood and pure air*

It has been shown that the nerves of *feeling* or *sensation*
run from the back portion of the spinal cord, and the nerves
of motion from its front portion.   They then are united in
the same cases, and are spread all over the body, thus united
whenever motion is required.   But the skin receives its
supply from the nerves of feeling alone, which are abundantly multiplied in a close net-work of nerves.   It is found
by experience that there is an intimate connection between
the exercise of the *nerves of motion* and the health of the
brain and other nerves, so that these may be regarded as
the *balance-wheel* of the whole nervous system.   The neglect
of the nerves of motion tends to produce a morbid sensitiveness of the other portions, while their appropriate action
yields vigor, quietude, and enjoyment to every other function.   Our Creator designed his creatures for industry and
activity, in gaining good for themselves and for their fellow-

beings, and to secure these a heavy penalty is affixed to inactivity of the muscular system.   Every other instrument
of the body becomes less susceptible to enjoyment, and more
sensitive to suffering in proportion to the use or neglect of
the nerves of motion.   From this we see the importance of
this next rule : *Take care that the health of the brain and
nerves is secured by the daily and abundant exercise of the
nerves of motion.*

The nerves of sensation, it has been shown, most abound
in the skin, while in their origin and branches they are intimately connected and bound up with the nerves of motion.
In this way the state of the skin influences very extensively
the whole nervous system, more so than any other bodily
organ.   Therefore, this rule is important: *Take care that
the health of the brain and nerves is secured by a proper attention to the health and cleanliness of the skin.*

It has been found by experience that the health and
strength of the brain and nerves is dependent on *sleep.*   In
this state the drain on the nervous fountain ceases, and it
has a season for accumulating its resources.   If there is not
enough time allowed for sleep, there is a slow draining of
nervous power which finally exhausts the nervous reservoir.
On the contrary, if too much time is given to sleep, the
system is exhausted by excess.   Seven hours of sleep is
the average, some require eight, and some but six.   Eight
hours of sleep is all that is needed by any healthy person,
and more than this tends to debilitate the nervous system.

Any excessive fatigue, either of body or mind, demands
an additional period of repose for the brain.   Persons who
use the brain a great deal, and under a strong pressure of
care and feeling, require extra periods for sleep.   This rule,
then, is important: *Take from six to eight hours of sleeep as
the general practice, but add more in cases of excessive activity
of mind or body.*

In many cases the health of the brain and nervous system demands *amusements.*   Any pursuit is an amusement
which is sought simply for the *present* pleasure it affords,
without reference to its future results.   Pleasure is a healthful stimulus to the brain and nerves, while anxiety, care,
and sorrow, have the opposite influence.   And no mind or

body can be a healthy one when every waking hour is devoted to what are the business and duties of life without intervening periods of recreation.

There are no amusements so useful as those that excite laughter. There are a set of nerves called the risible, and portions of the brain and body which are exercised by laughter. These the Creator designed should be used, and all who have attended most to physiology and the laws of health, declare that nothing is more promotive of good health than a hearty laugh. In every family some portion of every day should be devoted to social and domestic enjoyments, in which amusements should form a part.

So strong is the love of amusements, and especially of those that excite merriment, that there is danger of excess. This danger has led many conscientious persons to shun altogether what requires only to be taken in moderation. From a want of just views on this subject there has been too often a marked line of separation between those who seek amusements and those who avoid them—one class going to one extreme, and the other to the opposite. At the same time, those who seek amusement are usually the class who least need it, while those who most need recreations entirely avoid them. There is no nation in the world that give so much time to study, care, and business, with so little intervening amusements, as the Americans, and this is one reason of the general decay of health. This law, then, is important: *Let some portion of each day be allowed for recreation, especially by persons whose minds are burdenea by cares and duties.*

It is found that a simple *change of pursuits* has a healthful and refreshing influence on the brain, even when these pursuits are severe. This is owing to the fact that a different portion of the brain, and different sets of nerves, are called into action, allowing others to rest. It is found, also, that *regularity and system* have a great influence in lessening fatigue and care, so that a person that is systematic can accomplish far more labor, and with much less care, than can be done by one who has no such habits. This rule, then, is important: *Let there be change and variety in employments, and at the same time system and order.*

The brain can be made to suffer as severely from *inactivity* as from any other cause. The want of some noble and engaging pursuit in life, leaving all the faculties and affections without appropriate objects, is one of the most serious evils that is suffered by the wealthy and prosperous. The selfish pursuit of pleasure soon cloys, and the mind pines for something noble to relieve. And this longing is always proportioned to the amount of talent and sensibility of each mind. A small, or a phlegmatic, or a low and uncultivated mind, can more readily become reconciled to inactivity, or a life filled up with trifles.

But the higher a mind rises in the scale of being, the nobler the intellect and feelings, and the more cultivated the powers, the greater the suffering consequent on inactivity, and the greater the longing for high and noble objects of pursuit. The chief and grand law, then, of health for the brain and nerves is, *that all the powers and feelings of the mind be engaged in the pursuit of noble and benevolent objects.*

But the brain and nerves can be made to suffer severely, even when the intellect and feeling are engaged in noble pursuits, by an unbalanced and unequal exercise of the faculties and sensibilities. This may be seen in the case of some benevolent persons, who select some single department of benevolent effort to turn all their energies and feelings into that channel alone. Their domestic affections, their social duties, the enjoyments of taste, the relief of recreations, and many other departments of mental activity included in a well-balanced and well-developed mind, are neglected. In this way the character is deteriorated rather than improved, while the brain and nervous system suffer from an excess in one direction of activity, and from an equal neglect in another. Our Creator has given us no faculties of action or feeling which he did not design to have duly exercised in securing enjoyment to ourselves and to our fellow-beings. This, then, is an important law of health for the brain: *Take care that all the faculties and susceptibilities of the mind and body be duly exercised so as to secure a well-balanced mind in a healthful body.*

PART THIRD.

LETTER FOURTEENTH.

ABUSES OF THE BODILY ORGANS BY THE AMERICAN PEOPLE.

WE have noticed the construction of the most important organs of the human body, and the laws of health in the treatment of these organs. The next portion of the work will point out the methods by which the American people violâte these laws and thus bring disease, deformity, and death on themselves, and educate their children for the same sad experience. This will be done under the same heads as have been taken in the previous pages.

ABUSES OF THE BONES AND MUSCLES.

In another portion will be shown how the American people take such a course in regard both to diet and fresh air, that the bones and muscles are provided only with impure and unhealthy blood. In shops, manufactories, offices, counting-rooms, sleeping-rooms, sitting-rooms, churches, school houses, railroad cars, and almost every other place where human beings live, arrangements are made that, in nine cases out of ten, provide only impure air to breathe. Thus the capillaries of the bones and muscles never receive their proper supply of oxygen. This tends to make them weaker, softer, and smaller than they would be if nourished by blood properly oxygenized in the lungs.

At the same time the stomach, being loaded with an excess of food, and this food wrong in its selection, can not provide healthful chyle, and consequently there is a failure of proper nourishment for the bones and muscles.

It has been shown how much the health of the whole

system depends upon the proper and uniform action of all the muscles, and also that this exercise is most serviceable when the mind is at the same time interested in attaining some worthy object by this exercise.

Now the labor appointed to man in cultivating the earth, in preparing its fruits, and in many mechanical pursuits, will be found to be that which exercises all the muscles of the body appropriately and healthfully. So also the labor appointed to woman in the family state, involves just that variety of employment which, if wisely adjusted, would be exactly what is best calculated to develop every muscle most perfectly, while in the performance of these duties the mind has healthful occupation.

And yet every man who can do so, avoids these healthful pursuits as less honorable, and seeks in preference those that shut him up in study, office, or store, to overwork his brain and leave his muscular system to run down for want of vigorous exercise and fresh air. And so almost every woman, who has it in her power, turns off the work that would make herself and her daughters beautiful, graceful, and healthful, to hirelings, and takes sewing, reading, and other inactive pursuits as her exclusive portion.

By this method of dividing the labor of life, one portion of the world weaken their muscular system, either by entire inaction of both brain and muscle, or by the excess of brain-work and the neglect of muscular exercise. Another large portion, having all the work that demands physical exercise turned off upon them, overwork their bodies and neglect their brains. And almost the whole fail in the *equal* training of the muscular system, which alone secures that perfect development on which health and beauty so much depend.

Owing to the above causes, the great majority of the present generation have grown up with bones and muscles to a greater or less extent weaker, smaller, and less healthful, than their Creator designed they should be. His work has been marred and enfeebled by their own abuse and neglect, or by that of their parents or other ancestors.

Having thus prepared the bones and muscles by debility to yield readily to any injurious influences, a large majority of the mothers and daughters of the nation adopt a style of dress that is exactly calculated to produce disease and deformity.

In the first place, they dress the upper portion of the body so thin, that the spine and chest are exposed to sudden and severe changes of temperature in passing from warm to cold rooms, and this tends to weaken that portion. Then they accumulate such loads of clothing around the lower parts of the body, as debilitates the spine and pelvic organs by excess of heat. At the same time, they bind the ribs so tight, that there is a constant lateral pressure against one side of the spine, tending to produce a curvature that distorts one shoulder and one hip. At the same time the weight of clothing on the hips and abdomen presses down on the most delicate and important organs of life to move them from their proper positions, while pointed bodices, with whalebone pressure, co-operate as a lever in front, to accomplish the same shocking operation. The efforts of the Chinese mother in binding up her child's foot to distortion, is wisdom compared with the murderous folly thus perpetrated or tolerated by thousands of mothers and daughters in this Christian and enlightened age and nation. And the most terrible feature in this monstrous course is, that the evil thus achieved by a mother is often transmitted to her deformed offspring.

Besides these methods for distorting the muscles and bones others quite as effective are adopted.

Some children are made to sit still for hours on seats at school that do not properly support the body. Thus some of the muscles are debilitated, by over-exertion, to hold up the body, and finally failing, the discs of the spine are forced into the hardening process to supply the place of the muscles.

Other children are allowed to sit so many hours in wrong positions, either while reading or writing, as to bring on deformity by a similar process. Other children sleep on high pillows and in such uniformly wrong positions as induces deformity. Others are allowed to sit and stand in positions that lead to deformity.

Then again, when the evil results of these methods begin to develop, and the child is seen to be growing up with

crooked back, or projecting neck, or round shoulders, or all together, instead of ceasing the wrong treatment and securing
proper exercise, diet, and fresh air as the only true remedy,
braces are girt around the bones and muscles to increase the
very evil they are used to remedy.

Then, when it is discovered that *exercise* is needed for
a remedy, the habit is so suddenly invaded as to weaken
instead of giving strength. The slow and gradual change
would, indeed, meet the evil, but the sudden jerk only adds
to it. And then the plea is made that exercise is found by
trial to do more harm than good.

There is one mode of *exercise* that is very common, and is
earnestly defended on the ground of its healthful tendencies,
and that is *the dance*. There is no doubt that the Creator,
when he implanted that strong love of measured exercise to
the sound of music, intended that it should be gratified.
And were it the custom for families to go abroad into the
open air, in proper habiliments, at proper times, and dance
to the sound of music, and this were the only mode adopted,
it is probable that no such prejudice as now exists against
this amusement would have arisen. But how is the dance
usually conducted?

In the first place, it is commonly in the night season,
when quiet is better than exercise. Next, it is in rooms
where the air is vitiated by many lights and many breaths,
and where quiet is far better than a quickened circulation.
Next, the clothing of the female portion of the performers
is usually the very worst that could be selected for such an
occasion—too thin about the chest and too heavy below it.
Then, before the night is passed, the stomach, which should
rest when the muscles are exercised, is loaded with the most
unhealthful of all kinds of food, condiments, and drinks.
Finally, after the skin, stomach, and lungs have been debilitated by hours of abuse, and the whole brain and nervous
system exhausted by mental and physical excitement, the
company adjourn to cold halls and robing-rooms, and go
forth to ride through the night air, with weary, sleepy drivers, to weary, sleepy servants or friends, whom selfish amusements have deprived of proper repose and sleep. When
another generation has been trained to understand and obey

the laws of health, the beautiful and health-giving dance
will be rescued from its profanation and abuse. But in its
present state of degradation, entire abstinence is probably
the safest rule; for those who venture only a few steps will
probably be soon drawn far beyond their first intentions,
while their views of right and expediency will gradually sink
to the standard of their wishes, or yield to those of their
children.

ABUSES OF THE LUNGS.

It is the universally-acknowledged fact, that the present
generation of men and women are inferior in health and in
powers of endurance to their immediate ancestors. And in
all quarters the cause is sought, while many varying answers are given.

It is probable that no *one* cause can be assigned as the sole
reason. But it can be made to appear probable that the
abuse of the lungs by supplies of impure air has had more
influence than any one thing in the general decay of health.
Our ancestors always slept in cold and well-ventilated chambers. And in the family by day, the broad-mouthed chimney
and uncorked doors and windows secured a constant flow
of cool and pure air, while daily exercise in family work by
women and children, and out-door work by men and boys,
secured the cheerful spirits and healthful exercise most favorable to body and mind.

But as wealth and luxury have increasèd, houses have
been made tight, windows have been corked, fire-places
have been shut up, and close stoves and furnaces introduced.
Men work in heated counting-rooms, offices, stores, shops,
and manufactories, with brains stimulated and muscles inactive, or with both muscles and brains stimulated, while
the fetid effluvia of many skins and lungs accumulates as
the only fountain of supply to the lungs and the dependent
capillaries all over the body. Then they go home and sleep
with wives and children in close, unventilated, and sometimes heated rooms. And even when they travel, especially
in winter, when the cold and pure air would most invigorate,
they are packed in close cars, with a stove burning up the
oxygen and thinning the air, while windows are fastened

down and every crack made air-tight with frozen breaths. The idea that every pair of lungs needs a hogshead of pure air every hour as much as the stomach needs its daily food, is one that has never been acted on by one man in a thousand in arranging for his house, his place of business, and his family.

If society understood this subject as it will some day be considered, there would be health-officers to inspect every house in the land, and bring indictments for crime against every man that arranges to poison himself and his family by an unhealthful atmosphere.

One grand difficulty on this subject is, that the philosophy of ventilation has been so little attended to, practically, that not one in a thousand even of educated persons, not one in a hundred even of those who have studied physiology, and consider pure air as important to health, really know what is necessary to secure a proper ventilation.

The thing to be done is to secure a *gentle current* of air, which shall constantly pass in and out of a room or building where the lungs and skin of human beings are vitiating the atmosphere.

This being so, it is a very easy matter to ventilate any room, by simply having an opening at the top of one window and another at the top of a door. The size of this opening must be proportionate to the number of lungs that are to use the air. In a common-sized chamber, with two lodgers, an inch at the top of a window and an equal opening over the door, will ventilate sufficiently.

In ventilating a room, care must be taken that the current be not so large and so strong as to be sensibly felt by the inmates, as this will cause colds. There must be a gentle, imperceptible current established; and where a great deal of air is needed, to meet the wants of many inmates, several small openings must be made instead of any large one.

Churches and school-houses are best ventilated by furnaces placed under, and opening at one end of the room, while the ventilators at the top of the room should be at the opposite extremity. This makes a current pass through the whole house.

But if the furnace and ventilators are placed over each other, the current does not so entirely affect every part of the room, while the warm air passes off faster.

The collecting of large numbers of human beings in one building, to spend both day and night, always involves the gradual dilapidation of constitution to all, especially to the most susceptible, unless uncommon care is taken to provide a proper supply of pure air. All the rooms should open into long halls that are constantly swept by the outer air from opposite doors and windows. At the same time ventilators should open from each room to these halls, and then another opening be made to the outer air at the top of each window in every room.

But institutions could now be pointed out, where physiology has been taught for years, and yet where two or three hundred live, month after month, breathing chiefly impure air. In neither basement, kitchen, nor dining-hall, where the inmates perform daily exercises, are any *proper* arrangements for carrying off the impure air, vitiated by hundreds of lungs. School-rooms and lodging-rooms are equally unprovided with *proper* ventilation. Meantime the young inmates have their brain and nervous system on a constant drain by intellectual activity and moral responsibility. And then, as year after year, we hear that fevers and various diseases sweep off the young inmates by death, or send them home to recruit, their friends are all wondering what *can* be the reason there is so much sickness there!

So in our manufactories and shops of labor, thousands of the young congregate to labor in poisonous air, till their constitutions are undermined, and then return home to remain invalids for life.

To add to all the mischief of vitiated air, young women are generally girt so tight around the body, that the lower part of the lungs, where the air-cells most abound, are rarely used. *Abdominal breathing* has ceased among probably a *majority* of American women. The ribs also are girt so tight, in many cases, that even the *full* inspiration at the *top* of the lungs is impossible. And this custom has operated so, from parent to child, that a large portion of the female children now born have a deformed thorax, that has room only for imperfectly formed lungs. The full round chest of perfect womanhood is a specimen rarely seen, and every day diminishing in frequency.

To these abuses of the lungs are to be added the multiplied distortions caused by long-continued unnatural positions at school or at work, that cause round shoulders and bent forms, by which the lungs are cramped in size and action.

In many cases the attempt to ventilate rooms by ignorant or heedless persons is a serious evil. Such will wait till a room is hot, and its air almost poisonous, and then—when the skin of all its inmates is reeking with perspiration—open a door or window, and make a strong and direct draft, that, of course, causes colds and injurious chills. By this method many are so annoyed as to really hate ventilation and all its advocates.

The only proper and safe method is to have such arrangements made that a room is always perfectly ventilated at all times, and by such a process that no strong current is made in any direction. A window open at top, with a thin curtain over, on one side of a room, and another window or door, with a moderate opening, on the other side, suffices where there are few persons. When there are many, there must be a multiplication of the number of ventilating openings.

LETTER FIFTEENTH.

It has been shown that the health of the body is very dependent on the proper selection and proper amount of food.

In regard to the selection of food, it has been shown that there are these general classes:

First, animal and vegetable, which do not differ essentially in their constituents, both having exactly the same primary elements. The main respect in which they differ is, that animal food is more stimulating (not more nourishing) than vegetable, by which is meant that it tends to make all the organs of the body work faster. It is the predominance of *nitrogen* in animal food that gives it this stimulating quality.

Next, there is the *heat-forming* and the *flesh-forming* kinds of food. The heat-forming are those that supply most abundantly the carbon which is to combine with oxygen in the capillaries, and thus furnish fuel for the fires that cause animal heat. The stomach supplies the carbon to burn, and the lungs supply the oxygen to consume it. Butter, fat, oil, sugar, and molasses are the most prominent articles of this kind. The flesh-forming food is that portion which is most readily incorporated into the body as muscle, and does not furnish so large a proportion of carbon for animal heat. All kinds of grain, vegetables, and fruits, contain both the flesh-forming and the heat-forming ingredients. Indeed so do a greater portion of the articles of food. The classification relates only to the *predominance* of one or the other quality.

Next, there are the *nutritious* and *innutritious* kinds of food. The most nutritious are those that yield the largest quantity of nourishment in a given bulk. The innutritious food is that which is not assimilated into the body, but is useful, by bulk and stimulation, in forwarding the process of digestion. For food that is highly concentrated, so as to have a great deal of nourishment in a small bulk, does not digest alone so readily as when mixed with innutritive matter.

Finally, there are the *digestible* and *indigestible* kinds of food, which are classed with reference to the ease and speed with which they are carried through the process of digestion.

This account of the different kinds of food is recapitulated to show the philosophy of those laws of health that regulate *the selection of diet.* These rules indicate that knowledge, prudence, and discretion are needed in order to regulate the selection of food with reference to *climate, seasons, age, temperament, state of health,* and *nature of employments.* Those who live in a hot climate need a different diet from those living in a cold. The food of the summer should be modified from that of winter. The young should not eat some food that is suitable for the aged. Persons in one state of health, or with weak powers of digestion, should not take certain articles that are proper in other circumstances ; while persons who are engaged in sedentary employments may not take what would be safe to persons exercising constantly in the open air.

If the American people were a strong, hardy, unexcitable race like the German laborers that come among us, such rules for the selection of diet would be of less importance. But if it should appear that probably a majority of our people are either invalids or fast hastening to that condition, the matter becomes far more worthy of attention.

The course which has been pursued by a large number who have attempted to teach the public on this subject, has served greatly to embarrass and perplex. A great portion of such writers seem to be mounted on *hobbies.* Some advocate an exclusive vegetable diet, and in such an extravagant way as to make the impression that nothing is quite so bad for the human race as eating meat, and that most of the physical and moral evils of society would be ended by the adoption of a farinaceous and vegetable diet.

On the other hand, those who advocate a mixed diet, including animal food, write as if no man could become perfectly developed physically without meat. The impression is made that bread and vegetables, which really contain far more nourishment in a given bulk than any meat, is a *low* diet; that there is nothing that is so *nourishing* as a good piece of beef-steak; and that the poor creatures who have been kept for months on bread and butter, milk, fruits, and vegetables, must be "strengthened and built up" by porter, wine, and meat.

Then, again, certain articles of food will be hunted down as if in all cases and all circumstances they were rank poison; while others will be selected as good for all mankind in all circumstances.

But what is needed on this subject is, that the people should learn the construction of their own bodies, the nature of different kinds of food, and the laws that should regulate their selection, and then that they should use their judgment and common-sense in this as in all other matters. At the same time habits of self-control and principles of duty are needed to secure obedience to the dictates of discretion.   For want of all this, the great body of the American people are following a course which, in multitudes of cases, leads to certain disease, and shortens life.

In the animal kingdom there is no creature that does not succeed better than man in raising its young.   It is calculated that nearly one-third of the human race perish before they reach their third year; while no such mortality as this exists among the young of irrational animals.   We shall see the reasons for this, as we trace the various methods which are taken that are destructive to the health and life of young children.

In regard to the selection of food, there is no physician of any school but what allows that meat is more *stimulating* than any other food, and should be avoided whenever there are any tendencies to fevers or inflammation. All concede, also, that children are more excitable, and more liable to inflammatory attacks than grown persons. And yet the great mass of children in this country begin to eat meat the first and second year of life, which is the period of greatest danger from feverish and inflammatory attacks of all kinds. And it is often the case that meat is allowed twice, and sometimes thrice a day.

G

Little attention is paid to the peculiar temperament of children in regulating diet. A child of full habit that tends to inflammation, needs one course; while a child of thin blood, phlegmatic temperament, and slow movement, is safe with a diet that would destroy the other.

So in cold weather, a diet which is safe and proper may be very injurious in the heat of summer. As a general rule, children are safest and healthiest who eat little meat, little sugar, molasses, butter, and fats, and live chiefly on bread, milk, fruits, and vegetables.

This being so, the quantities of butter, molasses, and sugar heaped on to hot cakes—the meats, gravies, and fatty cooking—the stimulating condiments, and the candies and confectioneries that abound, are all so many sources of debilitation, disease, and death to the young.

In addition to this, children are allowed tea and coffee, which stimulate the nerves and brain, while the heat of these drinks tends to debilitate the stomach.

The adult population of our country pay little regard to the rules of prudence in selecting their food. Men of full habit and excitable nerves will eat meat and drink tea and coffee and other stimulating drinks, without the least knowledge or fear of the probable consequences. In summer meat and carbonaceous food is taken just the same as in winter, while the stimulating condiments are freely used. In our newer settlements, where most care and caution are important, meat at every meal, coffee twice or thrice a day, and hot bread, with other of the most indigestible kinds of cooking, abound; and in summer the same as in winter.

It is probable that a description of the most unhealthy and improper meal that could possibly be provided would include exactly what is found on the tables of a very large portion of, as it respects wealth, our most thriving population. And thus it is that the wear and tear on the constitution prepares the way for acute attacks that end life, or for chronic disease that beclouds all its enjoyments.

But the greatest evil is probably accomplished by the excesses in *quantity* of food. The great evil of condiments is not so much their influence on the circulation as the unnatural stimulation of appetite that they produce. This leads almost every person who uses them to take more food than the body demands, which overtaxes the system in throwing off the excess. In addition to this, the great variety of food which our country's abundance provides is another temptation to excess. Many persons eat after the appetite is satisfied simply to gratify the palate with some tempting viand.

The evils of excess in quantity of food are particularly injurious to children. The strength which would otherwise be employed in perfecting all their organs and functions is used up in relieving the system from the excess of needless food.

As a general fact, the more wealthy and prosperous a community becomes the more food and the less exercise is taken. To those who exercise a great deal in the open air there is less need of care, both as to selection and quantity of food; for the quickened circulation and good supply of oxygen meet the evil with less injury. But to those who have little air and little exercise the tempting varieties of the table, instead of a blessing, are a daily curse.

Here, however, there is need of caution in reference to books and papers that attempt to prescribe by weight how much every body should eat. Some persons require more food than others, and more is needed by the same person at one time than at another; and it is folly to guide all by one rule. If all will exercise enough, live in pure air, avoid stimulating condiments, and persevere in a plain and simple diet, *a healthy appetite* will return ; and this will be a steady and safe guide. Until this is secured, it is always safest to *stop before there is a sense of fullness and satiety*.

In regard to the *time* and *manner* of taking food, the Americans are celebrated for violating the rules of health.

In the first place, the rule requiring that there should be a period of rest to the brain and muscles before taking food is rarely regarded. Students and men of business rush to their noontide meal with brains throbbing with excitement and the circulation all disarranged. And the laboring classes do the same in reference to their excited muscular system. Both should allow half an hour of quiet to mind and body before setting the stomach to its labors.

In the same way the stomach is hurried in all its operations. Food is thrust into it half-masticated, and one bolus follows another before the needful process for each can be effected. Half an hour is the shortest time that should be allowed for a meal; and yet probably a majority of the busy workers of this nation do not allow much more than half this time.

Then, as soon as the stomach is thus improperly loaded, the brain, nerves, and muscles are all set to work again—thus drawing off the blood needed by the stomach to perform its digestive process.

Many persons, after eating their three meals a day, will load the stomach just before going to sleep, and thus keep up the labor of the system during its feeblest period, and when all its powers should rest.

Irregular periods of eating for children, and the candies and other confectionery so common in these days, are a prolific source of debility and disease. By these indulgences the stomach is taxed at all hours of the day, with short periods to rest. New food is constantly mixed up with that which is partially digested, while sweets of all kinds are the carbonaceous food that requires much exercise and much oxygen from the air to dispose of it safely. And yet it is city children and little pets, who seldom are allowed to romp in fresh air, that are most abundantly supplied with these pernicious articles.

Candies and sweet articles are highly concentrated nourishment that ought, when eaten, to be mixed with coarser food in order to secure proper digestion. This kind of food is more likely to turn acid on a weak stomach than any other, while none so surely tends to produce constipation.

An enormous abuse of the stomach and other digestive organs is from the quantities of quack medicines that are taken in this country; while the giving of *family* medicines by parents is scarcely less an abounding evil.

The grand objection to the taking of medicines, except when prescribed by a judicious and well-educated physician, is, that most of them are either poisonous substances or strong stimulants that strain all the animal economy to discharge them from the body; while their operation and re-

sults are matter of mere chance and *guess-work*. Whatever is put into the stomach is quickly taken into the circulation, and carried all over the body; and if it does
good in one point of the wonderfully complicated organs,
it may do as much harm to other portions.

Besides this, there are curious *chemical* changes going
forward in our bodies that none fully understand; and how
these medicinal agents will operate to produce new and
mischievous combinations no one can tell.

And yet men, women, and children, all over the land,
are pouring down medical liquids and pills to an incredible
extent; while vast fortunes are made by ignorant quacks
that, by lying advertisements, succeed in poisoning their
fellow-creatures by slow processes.

The abuse of the stomach, brain, and nerves by stimulating drinks, has become so terrible in this nation that the
whole country is roused to put an end to *one kind, i. e.,* the
alcoholic articles.

But the tea and coffee stimulants that are undermining
the constitutions of women and children, and the tobacco
smoking and chewing which is ruining the health or creat-
ing dangerous appetites for so many young men, still hold
their place even among conscientious and Christian people.
The light that drives away the demons of alcoholic stimulation, it is hoped, will gradually chase these kindred associates that hover over the feebler sex and helpless childhood.

ABUSES OF THE SKIN.

We have seen the curious construction of the skin, and
the important work it performs in regulating the heat of the
body, and in discharging through its required pores decayed
and poisonous matter that is drawn off by the veins and
lymphatics. *Twenty-eight miles* of perspiration tubes, all
lined with infinitely small capillaries, are placed all over the
skin, and through these *five-eighths* of the weight of daily
food and drink are discharged.

The decayed particles of the body accumulate on the
skin, and thus every portion of it needs to be washed *every
day*. And yet probably more than one half the American
people never wash *the whole body* from one end of the year

to the other; the face, neck, arms, and feet, being the only portions enjoying this privilege. Even a large part of those who occasionally wash the whole skin, do it only once a week, or perhaps once a month.

In this way, not only the skin itself becomes unhealthy, and less and less able to perform its functions, but the internal organs so intimately connected with it, become weak and disordered, being forced to do a portion of the duty that in a healthy state the skin would perform. The liver and the lungs are the special sufferers from this neglect and abuse.

The skin is a great sufferer from the methods taken by multitudes to keep it warm. The true method is to supply the blood of its capillaries with enough oxygen through the lungs, and to keep it in a healthy state by washing, friction, and exercise. When the blood-vessels are habitually filled with good, healthful blood, there is a warmth generated on the surface of the body, so that but little clothing is required. But just in proportion as the skin grows weak, and its capillaries imperfectly filled, there is a necessity for increasing the amount of clothing to prevent injurious chilliness.

Too much clothing tends to debilitate the skin; in the first place, by excess of warmth, next, by causing frequent perspiration when sitting in warm rooms, and finally, by excluding all access of the surrounding air. The unequal method of arranging the clothing of American women is a most fruitful cause of evil to the skin, as well as of diseases that have been referred to elsewhere. The upper portion of the body is dressed too thin, while the lower portion has such an excess gathered around it, as is a constant cause of debility to the skin as well as the internal organs. By this arrangement, on passing into cold rooms the upper portion of the skin is chilled, and the blood retreats to other parts of the body. Then when in warm rooms the lower portion of the body becomes excessively heated and debilitated by the consequent perspiration and warmth. The spinal cord, which is the parent of most of the nerves, is thus debilitated by chills in its upper portion and heat in its lower.

Instead of this, the whole body should be dressed very

nearly with the same amount of covering, except that the feet need more care than any other part. The reason of this is, that the circulation is slower in the extremities, and any interruption there affects the whole body more injuriously than in any other quarter. And yet there is no part of the person which fashion so much excludes from needful warmth and protection as the feet, especially among the most delicate and sensitive classes of the community. Multitudes of fashionable ladies, and the foolish women and young girls that imitate them, wear only a thin pair of hose and thin slippers in damp and cold weather, both in walking over cold floors and in the streets. Thus the circulation in the lower limbs is impeded, and the blood accumulates in the organs above to an unhealthful amount.

The skin also is abused both by neglect of ventilation and by the foolish methods taken to promote it. No part of the body suffers so much as the skin from a close, heated, and impure atmosphere. In this condition all its capillaries are deprived of the oxygen needed to purify the blood, while they are stimulated to excess, and debilitated by heat and perspiration.

Then some wiseacre will discover that the room needs ventilating, and open a window and door, which let in a current of cold air on to the skin at just the very time it is least able to bear it. Thus a cold is taken, and the sufferer is made to feel that all attempts to ventilate a room are folly and cruelty.

The skin is also abused by mistakes and excesses in bathing. A person unused to cold water should always commence its use with caution and moderation, beginning with tepid water in a temperate atmosphere, and increasing the cold as the skin and nerves gain strength. And the time and frequency of bathing should be regulated by the amount of animal heat and nervous power. Unaware of the need of these precautions, many persons injure the health of the skin and other organs by bathing in too cold water, or by practicing it too often or too long. The cold shower bath is a very strong and stimulating bath, and is not safe for children or for persons of a nervous or excitable temperament.

LETTER SIXTEENTH.

WE have seen that the brain and nerves are the organs by which the mind uses and controls the body, and that these are divided into various portions, each of which has its separate and peculiar work to perform. We have seen, too, that each brain has a nervous fountain for supplying the fluid which excites the nerves that stimulate every organ and function of the body. The capacities of this fountain vary with different persons, so that a degree of action to the brain and nerves which is perfectly safe and healthful to one, would entirely exhaust another.

We have seen that this nervous fountain may be exhausted by *excess* in the over-action of *any* of the powers of body or mind, and that the *equal* exercise of all our powers is indispensable to perfect physical and mental health, and to that happiness which is the result of perfect health.

Now every violation of any of the laws of health imposes a necessity for *unnatural* action to the brain and nerves, which tends to debilitate them and to diminish the fountain of nervous fluid. If the lungs inhale impure air, the brain suffers for its own diminished supply of oxygen, and it also suffers in being obliged to work unnaturally in ministering supplies of nervous fluid to those organs that must labor to remedy the evil. So also, if the stomach is loaded with an excess of food, or the kind of food is inappropriate to the wants of the body, the brain is taxed again in ministering extra supplies to the organs that must relieve the system. And so, again, if the skin is neglected, and thus restrained in its functions, the brain must labor to retrieve the evil.

Thus all violations of the laws of health are a drain on that central fountain which is the main reliance in what constitutes *a good constitution*.

We have seen, also, that the *nerves of motion* have a most important position in the system.   In order to impress this more strongly, here is a drawing which shows a small por-

Fig. 28.

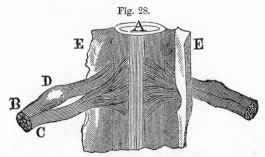

A the spinal marrow.   E a portion of its membrane, or skin, loosened to show the nerves.   D a nerve of sensation starting from one side of the spine.   C a nerve of sensation starting from the other side of the spine.   B the union of the two in one case.

Most of the branches from these trunks contain nerves of sensation and nerves of motion united in one case.

tion of the spinal marrow, with a pair of the nerves of motion and sensation branching on each side.   All the muscles have double nerves of this kind, one to *feel* and report to the brain, and the other to *move the muscles*.

Now it seems to be the office of the nerves of motion to *equalize* the nervous fluid and regulate its healthful flow to all portions of the system.   For this reason, inactivity of the muscles tends to an irregular and inharmonious flow of nervous energies, until finally there ceases to be a healthful and natural distribution of it.   From this results many of the strange and troublesome feelings that go by the general name of *nervousness*.

Such is the constitution of the brain, that the more the thoughts and feelings flow with great strength and for a long time in one direction, the more need there is for that equalization of the nervous fluid which muscular activity alone can secure.   And when this is withheld, the sensibility of the other portions of the brain is liable to become excessive, unnatural, and less under the control of the will.

These things being so, that vast portion of the American

people who sleep and live in badly ventilated rooms, who neglect to cleanse the skin, who eat bad food or take it irregularly and to excess, in the first place, *undermine their constitutions* by the extra taxation thus imposed on the brain and nerves. Then, in addition to this, multitudes are working the brain with cares, or labors, or study, or agitated feelings, without any of the equalizing influences that muscular activity would secure.

Thus the man of study or of business sleeps all night in bad air; then he goes to his office, store, or shop, with uncleansed skin to breathe bad air all day; then at his meals he takes meat, which is the most stimulating food, and condiments to stimulate appetite. These make him eat more than he needs, or he has such a variety as tempts to an overloaded stomach. Then he drinks tea, coffee, and perhaps alcohol, to stimulate the brain and nerves to increased action. Then he keeps tobacco in his mouth, to stimulate another portion of his brain. Then he stimulates the brain with anxiety, or business cares, or study, or deep thought all day long, without the relaxation of amusement or the refreshment of muscular exercise. And then at night he returns, exhausted, to sleep again in bad air, and next day renews the same exhausting process. Thus it is *stimulate, stimulate, stimulate the brain,* from year's end to year's end, till disease interrupts or death ends the career. Or, in other cases, the man becomes a pale, delicate, infirm being, every function and every organ ministering feebly to a half-living man. Thus it is that an active, vigorous, well-formed, healthy manhood is so rarely seen in this nation.

At the same time, a vast portion of the women of our nation are pursuing a course equally abusive of the brain and nervous system. As a general rule, woman originally is organized more delicately than the other sex, having a constitution that can not bear either labor or long or strong mental excitement as can the more vigorous sex. Then all her physical training is less invigorating than that of man. Then her pursuits, as a wife, mother, and housekeeper, are more complicated, less systematized, and less provided with well-trained assistants than the professions of men. American women have inherited from the English nation the notions of thrift, economy, industry, system, thoroughness, and comfort, which show so strongly in contrast to the habits of the lower classes of the Irish, German, and African races. And yet all their plans and efforts must be carried out mainly by poorly-trained menials of these nations.

Thus the larger portion of wives and mothers have the numberless and perplexing *cares* of nursery, kitchen, and parlor pressing on the brain from morning to night, while unsteady servants often leave them to perform heavy drudgeries for which neither strength nor training has prepared them. At the same time, the style of dress, and housekeeping, and the claims of social life also, are continually multiplying the complexity and number of domestic cares.

The hours in which the great majority of American mothers and housekeepers are *free from care*, and can go forth to breathe the pure air or join in social amusements, as is so common in other nations, come few and far between.

To this add all the mischief done by impure air, improper food, and neglect of the skin, which they share equally with the other sex.

But worst of all, add to these disadvantages the pernicious customs of dress, by which one half the body is subjected to extreme changes from heat to cold, while the other portion is compressed by tight girding, heated by accumulated garments, pressed downward by whalebones, and by heavy skirts resting over the most delicate organs.

Into our rural towns, even, these pernicious customs of dress have been carried by mantua-makers from the city, and still more by the miserable fashion-plates in our literature, that set forth the distortions of deformity and disease as models of taste and fashion.

In our country towns and among the industrial classes it will be found that the taxation of care and labor on the brain of women is even worse and greater than it is in the same class of our cities. The wives of rich farmers often are ambitious to carry out plans of labor and wealth with their husbands, while, at the same time, their daughters must be sent to boarding-school, and all the habits and tastes of city life must in consequence be mingled with other cares.

In former days, when women spun and wove, and made butter and cheese, their daughters were their intelligent and well-trained assistants; and the style of dress and all the details of life were simple, and easy, and comfortable. These days have passed away.

The great majority of American women have their brain and nervous system exhausted by too much care and too much mental excitement in their daily duties; while another class, who live to be waited on and amused, are as great sufferers for want of some worthy object in life, or from excesses in seeking amusement.

Our benevolent Creator designed his creatures to learn to live *out of themselves*, and for the good of their fellow-beings, and in this course to exercise their highest and noblest powers. Those who follow this design gain worthy objects to engage and interest all their higher faculties, and thus find true happiness. But the selfish, the indolent, and pleasure-seeking, soon learn that happiness is far from the path they pursue.

But the most melancholy view of all is, the course pursued in training the generation now coming on to the stage. In the first place, the children of over-taxed and over-excited parents come into being with an unnatural tendency to brain and nervous affections. It is probable that the *proportion* of children who are born with a vigorous and healthy constitution is smaller, in reference to the whole number born, than at any former period. This will be the more readily credited, when the statistics in regard to the. health of married women in a succeeding letter are examined.

Next, there never has been any previous generation of children who have been so extensively deprived of pure and cool air in nursery, school-room, and parlor, as those now on the stage. The air-tight stoves in bedrooms and sitting-rooms, the cooking stoves in kitchens, the close stoves in school-rooms, and the far greater care taken to make windows and doors tight, have secured this result.

Then the furnaces that are so generally used, keep the atmosphere of a house far warmer than it ever becomes with open fires. For when the body is warmed by *radiated* heat from a fire, the air never becomes so heated as when all warmth is to be gained from the surrounding atmosphere. And as the upper part of the room is always warmest, both stoves and furnaces keep the head warmer than the feet, and furnish to the lungs only a heated atmosphere to breathe.

In former days little girls took *cold* air baths all over their person whenever they went out. In these days, they are covered from all cool air, and they stand over *registers* and take *hot air baths* when they feel a chill or have cold feet.

Beside this, the school-rooms are made tighter and heated hotter than they ever could be in former days. At the same time, they are crowded with occupants whose brains, while struggling with bad air, are stimulated with intellectual drills and exciting motives to exertion, such as never were known to a former generation.

It is true, that much care has been taken in many cases to ventilate school-rooms. But the methods are such as usually entirely fail of the object aimed at. The fact that a school demands the entrance and discharge of a hogshead of fresh air every hour *for each one* of its fifty, one hundred, or two hundred pupils, is rarely made the basis of the arrangements for ventilation. But by far the greater portion of children suffer alternations of heat and cold made by poisonous and heated air at one time, diluted occasionally by currents of cold air from open doors or windows that come unequally, bearing deadly chills to the delicate pupils.

Little girls are especial sufferers in all that appertains to health. They must be housed most of the time in heated and impure air, and then when allowed to go abroad, they must wear thin slippers, and must not romp and run like the boys. And then, as they come to the most trying and critical period of life, the stimulation of brain increases, the exercise diminishes, and the monstrous fashions that bring distortion and disease are assumed.

In England, the higher classes rarely send a daughter to a boarding-school, but parents secure teachers to educate them at home, and take the greatest pains to secure a healthy and perfect physical development. But in this country, the greater portion of the wealthy classes send their daughters, at the most critical age, to be close packed in ill-ventilated chambers and school-rooms by night and by day, while all physical training is neglected, and the brain and nerves are stimulated by exclusive intellectual activity. Twenty years ago, a distinguished medical man gave it as his opinion that a majority of school girls had more or less of the curvature of the spine. A still more terrific deformity than this is now added as the result of our miserable neglect and abuse of the young.

In multitudes of families constituting the more wealthy classes, the following is a fair account of the manner in which the brain and nerves of young girls are trained to disease, and their bodies to deformity and suffering.

First, then, their brains struggle all night with impure blood in warmed and unventilated rooms. Then they dress with skins all polluted by the effluvia of the night, washing only the face and neck and arms. Next, they take strong tea and coffee to stimulate the brain and nerves, and then load the stomach with hot cakes, saturated with butter and sugar or molasses, or take stimulating animal food, done up in stimulating condiments. Next, they set the brain to work on school lessons, and then proceed to the close and crowded school-room, to tax the brain for hours with bad blood and intellectual labor.

Then comes a dinner of stimulating meat condiments and puddings or pies. Then three hours more of brain work in bad air. Then perhaps a solemn and decent walk around a few squares, and then the rest of the time, till the bed hour, is spent in a bad atmosphere, where a good part of the time study again taxes the brain. The tea hour also comes in to excite the nerves with another stimulating beverage.

Meantime all that art and fashion in dress can do to distort the bones, and misplace the most delicate organs, and interrupt every health function, is every day performed.

This is no imaginary picture, it is what is going on probably in the *majority* of families of the wealthy classes all over the land, both in city and country.

The work that Providence has appointed for woman in the various details of domestic life, is just that which, *if properly apportioned*, is fitted to her peculiar organization. If all the female members of a family divided all the labors of the cook, the nurse, the laundress, and the seamstress, so that each should have four or five hours a day of alternating light and heavy work, it would exercise every muscle in the body, and at the same time interest and exercise the mind. Then the remaining time could be safely given to intellectual, social, and benevolent pursuits and enjoyments.

But no such division is made. One portion of the women have all the exercise of the *nerves of motion*, and another have all the *brain-work*, while they thus grow up deficient and deformed, either intellectually or physically, or both. And so American women every year become more and more nervous, sickly, and miserable, while they are bringing into existence a feeble, delicate, or deformed offspring.

PART FOURTH.

LETTER SEVENTEENTH.

PERSONAL EXPERIENCE.

WE have attended to the most important organs of the human body, to the laws of health and happiness in the use of these organs, and to the neglect and abuses of them that are the most common. The next object will be to show the results of such abuses on the health and happiness of the American people.

It can immediately be seen that an attempt of this kind is a very difficult one. Every person's impressions on this subject must be based on the observations of one's own surrounding sphere, and any generalizing from a limited experience to that of a whole people, is liable to great inaccuracy and mistake.

In the present case, however, there have been data furnished by means of extensive, varied, and long-continued opportunities of observation which are unusual. But in order to present these data, some portion of my own experience is indispensable. It is the good aimed at, and the great evils to be remedied, that will prevail as a proper reason for this course.

All of my mother's eight children, who lived to maturity, through childhood bore the ruddy hue of perfect health, except myself, who received a delicate and scrofulous constitution—meaning by this term a tendency to humors in the blood. It was nearly two years from birth before I could walk, and the earliest memory of my life is sore eyes tied up to exclude light, and being dipped in the ocean to prevent rickets. This is mentioned to show the results of future physical training on a delicate child.

With a salary of only four hundred a year till his sixth child was born, and with only eight hundred till the eldest of thirteen was twenty, my father could never furnish his children any but the simplest fare and accommodations. The result was that we obeyed the laws of health, not from *principle*, but from *poverty*.

Tea and coffee were not provided for the young ones, and I never learned to love them till after maturity. When molasses was a dollar a gallon, and sugar fifty cents a pound, cakes and candies could not be afforded, while butter was always forbidden with meat. Stale bread, milk, vegetables, fruit, and plain-cooked meat, were the staples of diet.

As to fresh and pure air, we never had any other; for, with a house full of cracks and wide-mouth fire-places, it was impossible, either by day or night, that we could be stinted in this life-inspiring element.

As to clothing, one loose garment next the skin, a warm flannel petticoat in winter, with a woolen frock, shoes and stockings, were all that was worn in the house, and a shawl or overcoat was sometimes added in going outdoors. But oftener many hours were spent in the snow and ice without any added garment. No drawers around their limbs, in those days, interrupted the constant air-bath which every little girl received for her whole person.

As to exercise, the whole of childhood and youth, up to eighteen, was one long play-spell out of doors. In those days the "higher branches" had not invaded the school-room for girls. A quick and retentive memory secured all the lessons required in less than an hour of daily study, and a kindly teacher and easy parents looked with forbearance on school-hours spent in roving over hill and dale, and in concocting plays and jokes.

The result was that I can not recall the memory of a single day of sickness from infancy to the age of twenty. True, sometimes a cold was caught; and an anxious and tender father, on such occasions, would always summon the wise and good physician, known all over the State for his *great success* and *few doses*. His prescription, in the ver-

H

nacular and pronunciation of a century ago, shall here be preserved as a pleasing memorial of this good old friend. After placing the spectacles, and examining the pulse and tongue, this was the invariable response of my childhood's medical oracle:

"You may take a *tayspunful* of *Cramy* Tartar, and *power* on half a pint of *bilin* water, and *purt* in a piece of loaf-sugar about as big as a *hin's* egg, and a *leetle* orange peel, *jist* to give a pleasant flavor. and let her drink of it two or three times in the night, and I guess she'll be well in the morning." And the oracle's predictions were always fulfilled.

All the memories of my youth are those of *perfect* health, and that physical and mental enjoyment that are its natural attendants. Such was the result on a mind constitutionally a cheerful one, that the greatest trouble to me and to my parents was, that I was too happy and too merry to be able to think long of any thing solemn, or to fear any evil in this world or any other.

But when womanhood came, then I must earn my own livelihood. And so, after a period of preparation that shut me up in the house, I started as a teacher of music and painting, and thus was confined in the house to breathe such air as most young girls are condemned to inspire through all their school-life, generally both by night and day, especially at boarding-schools. In less than two years the weak eyes and cutaneous affections of infancy returned, proving that it was pure air and outdoor exercise that had protected me from them all through my childhood and youth.

Next came sorrow—the heaviest and bitterest, and then religion, with its solemn realities, urging new and heavy responsibilities. Then, at the age of twenty-three, the institution was commenced that, for ten years, employed every energy. During most of that time, as principal of an institution numbering from one hundred to one hundred and sixty scholars, the larger portion boarding pupils, there was an amount of labor, excitement, responsibility, and care involved, such as kept the brain and nervous system on a constant stretch.

During the latter part of that period, in addition to the cutaneous difficulty, an affection was manifested which then was unintelligible, but which, with present knowledge, is easily explained. It was a singular susceptibility of the nervous system to any slight wound, bruise, or sprain. Such slight accidents would bring on an affection in the injured part, which was a semi-paralysis of the nerves of motion, attended by an extreme sensitiveness of the whole nervous system, while the injured limb remained weak and nearly useless for from two to twelve months. At first these attacks gradually passed away, but finally the sciatic nerve of one limb seemed to become permanently weakened, while, as a sort of barometer of health, its strength rose or fell as the general health sunk or rose. With the knowledge now gained by long and varied experience, one single prescription would, it is believed, have furnished the remedy for infirmities of twenty years' continuance. It would have been simply this: "Take a great deal of exercise; breathe only pure air, both by day and night; bathe often; never exercise the brain more than five or six hours a day; relinquish all carbonaceous articles of diet; and never exercise the weak limb beyond its relative strength."

But all these rules were habitually violated without any knowledge of the consequent results. And yet during that whole period, I was constantly under the care of the most celebrated regular physicians of Connecticut, Massachusetts, or Ohio. Yet not one of them ever inquired in regard to the ventilation of my sitting or sleeping rooms, nor the amount of exercise taken, nor the nature of my food, nor directed the bathing of the skin, nor told me to save the weak limb from any excess of exercise.

The history of my medical experience under talented, highly-educated, and celebrated physicians, is worthy of attention and reflection.

For the cutaneous difficulty various washes and drugs were recommended, which never made any impression. One very celebrated physician directed a *teaspoonful* of sulphur *before every meal for five or six months*. This was obeyed without any good result. As before stated, this affection commenced when outdoor exercise ceased and confinement to school commenced, about at the age of nineteen. At the termination of school-teaching, and at a period when outdoor life was measurably resumed, a friend suggested the relinquishing of all carbonaceous food, not from any scientific knowledge, but because *some one* was once thus cured. The experiment was tried, and with entire success.

But the sensibility of the nervous system increased every year of school-life, and the semi-paralysis attacks multiplied in frequency and duration. The grand remedy tried for this was *carbonate of iron*, which I was directed to take at the rate of *a heaping teaspoonful before every meal*, and this was continued month after month by direction. I think in all my various attacks I must have taken not less than a bushel-measure of this article.

On one occasion, when, by two successive accidents, both a hand and a foot were rendered useless, an eminent surgeon and physician tried severing the wounded nerves from their centres, but with no good result.

By advice of another physician the whole spine was covered with *tartar emetic pustules* for several weeks, without any result but evil.

Finally, after ten years of school-teaching, the nervous fountain gave out entirely. I could neither read, write, or converse, nor even bear to hear conversation. From sheer inability to do any thing else, I was driven to journeying about to visit friends.

During the time of my boarding-school experience, I usually attended any pupils who were sick, in company with the physician. After a while, I found that in almost every case the prescription was "calomel and jalap." And, as I now remember, these were all cases where young girls were shut up from fresh air and exercise, and in which I now suppose that one or two days of fasting, the stopping of all carbonaceous food, and a good deal of pure, cool air by day and night, with bathing the skin, together with a proper amount of muscular exercise, would have been the true remedy.

During the subsequent years of traveling and visiting, medical men of reputation were consulted in every section. Every function of life was proceeding in perfect order; every organ seemed in entire health; what could be the cause of this nervous excitability centring, as it usually did, in one limb? Again the regular practitioners tried their skill. One distinguished physician was confident the disease arose from the stomach; and so, though not a symptom of any trouble came from that quarter, dose after dose was administered for that organ.

Next galvanism was prescribed, but without effect. Next the new school of homœopathy was invoked, and a shower of innocent little pellets were poured into the stomach, all to no purpose. Next I encountered Dr. Buchanan and his theory of *Neurology*, of which some account will be given in a note at the end. This experience produced a strong impression in reference to future probable discoveries of the remedial agency of *animal magnetism*.

Not a long time after, a very learned professor urged my visiting a *clairvoyant*, who had performed wonderful cures, and who, he felt sure, could benefit my weak limb. My visit to her still more impressed me with the probable efficacy of animal magnetism in discovering and remedying disease. But in my case her prescriptions of Sherwood's Electro-Magnetic Machine, and some "bitters for the stomach," were of no avail. Next, on visiting at the West, I encountered a lecturer on *Psychology*, who assured my brother that my case could be cured by his method. And so I sat and stared for some fifteen minutes at a silver sixpence held in my hand, and then my brother stroked me and stared at me—and this day after day, but all to no purpose.

Next I encountered a most remarkable clairvoyant, some of whose performances will also be detailed in the above-mentioned note. But all her wonderful powers were baffled by my case.

Soon after this the *Water Cure* came to my knowledge, and I spent nearly a year at the most celebrated establishment for this treatment. I was duly questioned, and learning that I once had suffered from a cutaneous difficulty, it was clear to my physician that all my trouble of the nerves arose from "humors in the blood." And so all the water-engines were set in full play to wash them out. In the first place a gradual process was pursued on one then so weak as to be scarcely able to walk with two supporters. But after some three or four weeks this was the detail of my treatment:

At four in the morning packed in a wet sheet; kept in it

from two to three hours; then up, and in a reeking perspiration immersed in the coldest plunge-bath. Then a walk as far as strength would allow, and drink five or six tumblers of the coldest water. At eleven A.M. stand under a douche of the coldest water falling *eighteen feet, for ten minutes.* Then walk, and drink three or four tumblers of water. At three P.M. sit half an hour in a *sitz* bath (*i. e.* sitting bath) of the coldest water. Then walk and drink again. At nine P.M. sit half an hour with the feet in the coldest water, then rub them till warm. Then cover the weak limb and a third of the body in wet bandages, and *retire to rest.* This same wet bandage to be worn all day, and kept constantly wet.

For three months this method was pursued, the doctor and patient all the time looking for "a crisis" that should bring out the "bad humors." At last a boil was developed, the brilliant harbinger, it was hoped, of many more. But none ever came after, nor could any "skin crisis" be made to appear that at all met the demands of the physician. At last, after more than a year of persevering efforts, the theory of "humors in the blood," as the cause of the nervous debility, seemed to be on the wane.

Soon after, another establishment was visited by quite a number of the most intelligent of my fellow-patients, who reported wonderful cures by a man who detected disease by a peculiar magnetic power in the ends of his fingers. As a matter of curiosity I joined them, was examined, and found that the cause of my weak limb was "an accumulation of mucus on the coats of the lower intestines." Willing to try an experiment which I felt sure could do no harm (for in all this drenching and drinking I certainly gained rather than lost strength), I directed the doctor to muster his engines and try his skill. For six weeks he labored to bring on a "mucus crisis," when suddenly he departed this life, and I departed this kind of treatment, at least so far as to give up the hope of a cure on the "mucus theory."

In this last institution I observed that the severity of the water treatment was considerably reduced, and yet there seemed to be greater success.

Next I resided for six months in a Water Cure where the treatment was still more mild, and yet such results were witnessed as strengthened the conviction that the heroic treatment, as it was called, was not fitted for the excitable and debilitated American constitution. After that I resided at intervals in several other Water Cures, chiefly for the benefit of friends, or for purposes of inspection.

Finally, I was led to reside in an institution where the main reliance was placed on *exercise*, in connection with a strict obedience to *all* the laws of health. My interest was awakened in this direction by works published in France and England, which were put into my hands by a distinguished female physician (Miss Elizabeth Blackwell, of New York city), who spent several years in the best medical schools of Europe in acquiring her profession.

In these volumes I became acquainted with the system of the distinguished Swedish philanthropist *Ling*. The orphan son of a poor clergyman, he was first distinguished by his genius and perseverance in acquiring a superior education on the most liberal scale. Being afterward employed as master of fencing, he took up the profession in a scientific view, and directed special attention to anatomy, physiology, and connected sciences, in order to perfect a system of exercises in harmony with nature. He assumed the principle of never adopting any movement till he could detect its exact effects on the whole organism, and apply it to use scientifically. By this process he finally evolved a system which aims in the first course to develop equally and perfectly the whole human form, and in the second place to remedy both deformity and disease.

After many years of trial and persevering efforts, this humble youth became distinguished at the court of Sweden as a public benefactor. He was knighted, and appointed professor and head of a public institution for preparing teachers to propagate his system. Several years ago it was thus introduced into all military academies, universities, colleges, town-schools, country-schools, and orphan-asylums of Sweden. And such were the results that the system has been carried into several other European nations under the authority of their governments.

In visiting the Health Establishment where exercise was the main reliance for the cure of disease, one great aim was to ascertain whether the system was scientific or empirical, and whether it was taken from Ling as a whole or in part.

During two months' residence in that institution, such results were witnessed as were entirely satisfactory as to the curative power of a well-directed system of *curative exercises*, even where it was not scientific, but empirical. In this case neither medicine nor water-treatment were relied upon, but strict obedience to the laws of health, and a system of vigorous exercise, commenced moderately, and increased daily till the nervous and muscular system were brought up to a tone and power which seemed wonderful, especially in a community of chronic invalids.

Of course a personal trial was made of its efficacy; and as one result it may be mentioned that, in the space of six weeks, the exercises designed to strengthen' my lungs so expanded the chest as to make it necessary to enlarge all the clothing two inches around the waist, and three inches across the chest. At the same time a degree of general vigor was gained that had not been experienced for years, and the weak limb seemed to gain more than from any previous method of treatment.

But at a time when there seemed to be a fair prospect of an entire cure by this treatment, by the carelessness of an employé of a railroad, I was thrown down, and dragged by a car in motion, and nearly thrown under the wheels. The fright, the jar, and the strain on a weakened limb, brought on a nervous attack, which disabled me for a whole year. And until this time the effects have not so ceased as that a fair trial can again be made of this method of exercise.

Thus, during a period of ten or twelve years, I have resided as a patient or boarder at not less than *thirteen* different health establishments, while, in my extensive journeys and visits, I have come into the sphere of almost every kind of medical treatment, either by my own experience or by that of my intimate friends. I have also resided at different periods in all the Free States.

In the following letters will be presented some of the results thus obtained.

LETTER EIGHTEENTH.

STATISTICS OF FEMALE HEALTH.

DURING my extensive tours in all portions of the Free States, I was brought into most intimate communion, not only with my widely-diffused circle of relatives, but with very many of my former pupils who had become wives and mothers. From such, I learned the secret domestic history both of those I visited and of many of their intimate friends. And oh! what heartaches were the result of these years of quiet observation of the experience of my sex in domestic life. How many young hearts have revealed the fact, that what they had been trained to imagine the highest earthly felicity, was but the beginning of care, disappointment, and sorrow, and often led to the extremity of mental and physical suffering. Why was it that I was so often told that "young girls little imagined what was before them when they entered married life?" Why did I so often find those united to the most congenial and most devoted husbands expressing the hope that their daughters would never marry? For years these were my quiet, painful conjectures.

But the more I traveled, and the more I resided in health establishments, the more the conviction was pressed on my attention that there was a terrible decay of female health all over the land, and that this evil was bringing with it an incredible extent of individual, domestic, and social suffering, that was increasing in a most alarming ratio. At last, certain developments led me to take decided measures to obtain some reliable statistics on the subject. During my travels the last year I have sought all practicable methods of obtaining information, and finally adopted this course with most of the married ladies whom I met, either on my journeys or at the various health establishments at which I stopped.

I requested each lady first to write the *initials* of *ten* of the married ladies with whom she was best acquainted in her place of residence. Then she was requested to write at each name, her impressions as to the health of each lady. In this way, during the past year, I obtained statistics from about two hundred different places in almost all the Free States.

Before giving any of these, I will state some facts to show how far they are reliable : In the first place, the *standard of health* among American women is so low that few have a correct idea of *what a healthy woman is*. I have again and again been told by ladies that they were " perfectly healthy," who yet, on close inquiry, would allow that they were subject to frequent attacks of neuralgia, or to periodic nervous headaches, or to local ailments, to which they had become so accustomed, that they were counted as "nothing at all." A woman who has tolerable health finds herself so much above the great mass of her friends in this respect, that she feels herself a prodigy of good health.

In the next place, I have found that women who enjoy universal health are seldom well informed as to the infirmities of their friends. Repeatedly I have taken accounts from such persons, that seemed singularly favorable, when, on more particular inquiry, it was found that the greater part, who were set down as perfectly healthy women, were habitual sufferers from serious ailments. The delicate and infirm go for sympathy, not to the well and buoyant, but to those who have suffered like themselves.

This will account for some very favorable statements, given by certain ladies, that have not been inserted, because more accurate information showed their impressions to be false. As a general fact, it has been found that the more minute the inquiry, the greater the relative increase of ill health in all these investigations.

Again, I have found that ladies were predisposed usually to give the *most favorable* view of the case ; for all persons like to feel that they are living in " a healthy place" rather than the reverse.

Again, I have found that almost every person in the result obtained, found that the case was worse than had been supposed, the proportion of sick or delicate to the strong and healthy being so small.

It must be remembered, that in regard to those marked as "sickly," "delicate," or "feeble," there can be no mistake, the knowledge being in all cases *positive*, while those marked as "well" may have ailments that are not known. For multitudes of American women, with their strict notions of propriety, and their patient and energetic spirit, often are performing every duty entirely silent as to any suffering or infirmities they may be enduring.

As to the terms used in these statements, in all cases there was a previous statement made as to the sense in which they were to be employed.

A "perfectly healthy" or "a vigorous and healthy woman" is one of whom there are *specimens* remaining in almost every place; such as used to *abound* when all worked, and *worked in pure air*.

Such a woman is one who can through the whole day be actively employed on her feet in all kinds of domestic duties without injury, and constantly and habitually has a feeling of perfect health and perfect freedom from pain. Not that she never has a fit of sickness, or takes a cold that interrupts the feeling of health, but that these are out of her ordinary experience.

A woman is marked "well" who usually has good health, but can not bear exposures, or long and great fatigue, without consequent illness.

A woman is marked "delicate" who, though she may be about and attend to most of her domestic employments, has a frail constitution that either has been undermined by ill health, or which easily and frequently yields to fatigue, or exposure, or excitement.

In the statements that follow, I shall place first those which are *most reliable*, inasmuch as in each case personal inquiries were made and the specific ailments were noted, to show that nothing was stated without full knowledge. As a matter of delicacy, the *initials* are changed, so that no individual can thus be identified.

MOST RELIABLE STATISTICS.

Milwaukee, Wis. Mrs. A. frequent sick headaches. Mrs. B. very feeble. Mrs. S. well, except chills. Mrs. L. poor health constantly. Mrs. D. subject to frequent headaches. Mrs. B. very poor health. Mrs. C. consumption. Mrs. A. pelvic displacements and weakness. Mrs. H. pelvic disorders and a cough. Mrs. B. always sick. Do not know one perfectly healthy woman in the place.

Essex, Vt. Mrs. S. very feeble. Mrs. D. slender and delicate. Mrs. S. feeble. Mrs. S. not well. Mrs. G. quite feeble. Mrs. C. quite feeble. Mrs. B. quite feeble. Mrs. S. quite slender. Mrs. B. quite feeble. Mrs. F. very feeble. Knows but one perfectly healthy woman in town.

Peru, N. Y. Mrs. C. not healthy. Mrs. H. not healthy. Mrs. E. healthy. Mrs. B. pretty well. Mrs. K. delicate. Mrs. B. not strong and healthy. Mrs. S. healthy and vigorous. Mrs. L. pretty well. Mrs. L. pretty well.

Canton, Penn. Mrs. R. feeble. Mrs. B. bad headaches. Mrs. D. bad headaches. Mrs. V. feeble. Mrs. S. erysipelas. Mrs. K. headaches, but tolerably well. Mrs. R. miserably sick and nervous. Mrs. G. poor health. Mrs. L. invalid. Mrs. C. invalid.

Oberlin, Ohio. Mrs. A. usually well, but subject to neuralgia. Mrs. D. poor health. Mrs. K. well, but subject to nervous headaches. Mrs. M. poor health. Mrs. C. not in good health. Mrs. P. not in good health. Mrs. P. delicate. Mrs. F. not in good health. Mrs. F. not in good health.

Wilmington, Del. Mrs. ——, scrofula. Mrs. B. in good health. Mrs. D. delicate. Mrs. H. delicate. Mrs. S. healthy. Mrs. P. healthy. Mrs. G. delicate. Mrs. O. delicate. Mrs. T. very delicate. Mrs. S. headaches.

New Bedford, Mass. Mrs. B. pelvic diseases, and every way out of order. Mrs. J. W. pelvic disorders. Mrs. W. B. well, except in one respect. Mrs. C. sickly. Mrs. C. rather delicate. Mrs. P. not healthy. Mrs. C. unwell at times. Mrs. L. delicate. Mrs. B. subject to spasms. Mrs. H. very feeble. Can not think of but one perfectly healthy woman in the place.

Paxton, Vt. Mrs. T. diseased in liver and back. Mrs. H. stomach and back diseased. Mrs. W. sickly. Mrs. S. very delicate. Mrs. C. sick headaches, sickly. Mrs. W. bilious complaints. Mrs. T. very delicate. Mrs. T. liver complaint. Mrs. C. bilious sometimes, well most of the time. Do not know a perfectly healthy woman in the place. Many of these are the wives of wealthy farmers, who *overwork* when there is no need of it.

Crown Point, N. Y. Mrs. H. bronchitis. Mrs. K. very delicate. Mrs. A. very delicate. Mrs. A. diseased in back and stomach. Mrs. S. consumption. Mrs. A. dropsy. Mrs. M. delicate. Mrs. M. G. delicate. Mrs. P. delicate. Mrs. C. consumption. Do not know one perfectly healthy woman in the place.

Batavia, Illinois. Mrs. H. an invalid. Mrs. G. scrofula. Mrs. W. liver complaint. Mrs. K. pelvic disorders. Mrs. S. pelvic diseases. Mrs. B. pelvic diseases very badly. Mrs. B. not healthy. Mrs. T. very feeble. Mrs. G. cancer. Mrs. N. liver complaint. Do not know one healthy woman in the place.

Oneida, N. Y. Mrs. C. delicate. Mrs. P. scrofula. Mrs. S. not well. Mrs. L. very delicate and nervous. Mrs. L. invalid. Mrs. L. tolerably well. Mrs. A. invalid. Mrs. W. broken down. Mrs. D. feeble. Mrs. W. pale but pretty well.

North Adams, Mass. Mrs. R. scrofula and liver complaint. Mrs. R. consumption. Mrs. C. consumption. Mrs. B. liver complaint. Mrs. B. consumption. Mrs. B. general debility. Mrs. F. consumption. Mrs. W. paralytic. Mrs. W. confined always to her bed. Mrs. R. scrofula.

Charlotte, Vt. Mrs. W. spinal complaint. Mrs. D. spinal complaint. Mrs. N. spinal complaint. Mrs. R. bilious and paralytic. Mrs. R. pelvic disorders. Mrs. H. heart disease and dropsy. Mrs. B. dropsical. Mrs. H. pelvic disease and palsy. Mrs. H. scrofula and consumption. Mrs. S. quite delicate. Knows but one perfectly healthy woman in the place.

Maria, N. Y. Mrs. H. consumption. Mrs. E. dyspepsia. Mrs. T. dyspepsia. Mrs. D. consumption. Mrs. P. dyspepsia. Mrs. R. sickly. Mrs. M. sickly. Mrs. R. delicate. Mrs. S. sickly. Mrs. R. consumption. Knows not one perfectly healthy woman in the place.

Vergennes, Vt. Mrs. L. delicate. Mrs. H. consumption. Mrs. H. consumption. Mrs. C. sickly. Mrs. S. liver complaint. Mrs. S. asthma. Mrs. S. sickly. Mrs. B. bronchitis. Mrs. S. consumptive. Mrs. B. delicate. Does not know a perfectly healthy woman in the place.

Brooklyn, N. Y. Mrs. B. very delicate. Mrs. G. scrofulous.

Mrs. R. pelvic displacements. Mrs. I. nervous headaches. Mrs. A. pelvic diseases. Mrs. W. heart disease. Mrs. S. organic disease. Mrs. B. well but delicate. Mrs. L. well but delicate. Mrs. C. delicate.

Berlin, Conn. Mrs. A. dyspepsia. Mrs. B. quite delicate. Mrs. C. nervous headaches. Mrs. G. pelvic disorders. Mrs. M. weak lungs. Mrs. F. not sound. Mrs. C. delicate. Mrs. N. vigorous and healthy. Mrs. C. well. Mrs. A. delicate.

Whitestown, N. Y. Mrs. A. consumptive. Mrs. P. well but delicate. Mrs. M. well but delicate. Mrs. S. pelvic disorders. Mrs. R. dropsy. Mrs. B. pelvic disorders. Mrs. H. sick headaches. Mrs. K. organic disorder. Mrs. B. well but delicate. Mrs. T. bronchitis.

Proctorville, Vt. Mrs. B. well. Mrs. H. well. Mrs. S. pelvic and stomach disorders. Mrs. S. not healthy. Mrs. F. not healthy. Mrs. B. sickly. Mrs. C. not healthy. Mrs. W. not healthy. Mrs. A. vigorous and usually well. Knows no other strong and healthy woman.

Saratoga, N. Y. Mrs. M. pelvic disorders. Mrs. H. pelvic disorders. Mrs. A. pelvic disorders. Mrs. C. well. Mrs. C. neuralgia. Mrs. P. well. Mrs. T. consumptive. Mrs. J. tolerably well. Mrs. B. consumptive. Mrs. B. not well. Knows only one more well one among her acquaintance.

Saratoga, N. Y. (by another resident). Mrs. T. pelvic disorder. Mrs. C. pelvic disease. Mrs. H. not well. Mrs. S. well and strong. Mrs. B. tolerably well. Mrs. M. usually well. Mrs. O. headaches. Mrs. H. O. well. Mrs. S. delicate. Mrs. P. not well.

Canandaigua, N. Y. Mrs. A. well. Mrs. B. an invalid. Mrs. C. delicate. Mrs. H. delicate. Mrs. H. an invalid. Mrs. J. well. Mrs. P. delicate. Mrs. A. well. Mrs. C. an invalid. Mrs. W. well.

Livonia, N. Y. Mrs. H. rheumatic. Mrs. R. healthy and vigorous. Mrs. S. well. Mrs. R. good health. Mrs. P. very poor health. Mrs. B. well. Mrs. G. an invalid. Mrs. S. delicate. Mrs. T. poor health. Mrs. ——, pelvic disorders.

Turkhannock, Penn. Mrs. P. delicate and sickly. Mrs. L. delicate and well. Mrs. R. well and vigorous. Mrs. S. tolerably well. Mrs. C. well. Mrs. S. healthy. Mrs. T. consumption. Mrs. M. healthy. Mrs. R. well. Mrs. ——, pelvic disorders.

Bath, N. Y. Mrs. H. an invalid. Mrs. H. rheumatic. Mrs. H.

healthy and vigorous. Mrs. S. vigorous. Mrs. K. delicate. Mrs. K. very healthy. Mrs. W. broken down. Mrs. W. tolerably well. Mrs. W. an invalid. Mrs. H. poor health.

Castleton, N. Y. Mrs. S. sickly. Mrs. W. healthy. Mrs. S. very delicate. Mrs. H. delicate. Mrs. H. delicate. Mrs. B. delicate. Mrs. W. not healthy. Mrs. H. not healthy. Mrs. D. not healthy.

The following were furnished by ladies who simply arranged the names of the ten married ladies best known to them in the place of their residence, in three classes, as marked over the several columns:

Residence.	Strong and perfectly Healthy.	Delicate or Diseased.	Habitual Invalids.
Hudson, Michigan	2	4	4
Castleton, Vermont	Not one.	9	1
Bridgeport, "	4	4	2
Dorset, "	Not one.	1	9
South Royalston, Mass....	4	2	4
Townsend, Vermont......	4	3	3
Greenbush, New York....	2	5	3
Southington, Connecticut.	3	5	2
Newark, New Jersey.....	2	3	5
New York City	2	4	4
Oneida, New York	3	2	5
Milwaukee, Wisconsin....	1	3	6
Rochester, New York.....	2	6	2
Plainfield, New Jersey....	2	4	4
New York City	3	6	1
Lennox, Massachusetts...	4	3	3
Union Vale, New York...	2	5	3
Albany, " ...	2	3	5
Hartford, Conn.	1	5	4
Cincinnati, Ohio.........	1	4	5
Andover, Mass...........	2	5	3
Brunswick, Maine	2	5	3

Residence.	Strong and Healthy.	Delicate or Diseased.	Invalids.
Southington, Connecticut.	3	5	2
Rochester, New York.....	2	6	2
Albany, "	2	4	4
Milwaukee, Wisconsin....	1	3	6
Plainfield, New Jersey ...	2	4	4
New York City	3	6	1
New York City	2	4	4
Worcester, Massachusetts.	1	6	2
Newark, New Jersey	2	3	5
Bonhomme, Missouri.....	3	5	2
Painted Post, New York..	1	3	6
Wilkins, " ..	2	3	5
Johnsburg, " ..	3	6	1
Burdett, " ..	4	3	3
Horse Heads " ..	3	2	5
Pompey " ..	4	4	2
Tioga, Pennsylvania	3	4	3
Lodi, New York..........	2	5	3
Seymour, Connecticut....	3	7	0
Williamsville, New York..	4	2	4
Herkimer, " ..	3	2	5
Hudson, Michigan	2	4	4
Kalamazoo, "	3	6	1

The following are those not so reliable as the preceding, as the papers were some of them not clear, and some uncertainty about others for want of personal inquiry:

Cattskill, N. Y. Three vigorous, two well, three delicate, two sickly.

Batavia, N. Y. One vigorous, two well, three delicate, one sickly.

Ogden, N. Y. Three well, five well but delicate, two sickly.

Utica, N. Y. Nine well but not vigorous, one invalid.

Rhinebeck, N. Y. One vigorous, six well but not vigorous, one delicate, one invalid.

Cooperstown, N. Y. Two vigorous, five well, two delicate, two sickly.

Lima, N. Y. Five well, three delicate, two sickly.

Rockaway, N. Y. Two vigorous, five well, one delicate, two sickly.

Brockport, N. Y. Three vigorous, six well, one delicate, one sickly.
Buffalo, N. Y. Five well, five delicate.
Potsdam, N. Y. Eight tolerably well, two sickly.
Rome, N. Y. Two well, seven tolerably well, one sickly.
Rochester, N. Y. Four well, three delicate, three sickly.
Princeton, N. J. Four well, five well but delicate, three sickly.
Muncy, Penn. Two vigorous, six well but delicate, two sickly.

The remainder of accounts furnished being less reliable, for want of opportunities of definite inquiry on my part, and will therefore be omitted. But they do not essentially differ from these presented.

I will now add my own personal observation. First, in my own family connection: I have nine married sisters and sisters-in-law, all of them either delicate or invalids, except two. I have fourteen married female cousins, and not one of them but is either delicate, often ailing, or an invalid. In my wide circle of friends and acquaintance all over the land out of my family circle, the same impression is made. In Boston I can not remember but one married female friend who is perfectly healthy. In Hartford, Conn., I can think of only one. In New Haven, but one. In Brooklyn, N. Y., but one. In New York city, but one. In Cincinnati, but one. In Buffalo, Cleveland, Chicago, Milwaukee, Detroit, those whom I have visited are either delicate or invalids. I am not able to recall, in my immense circle of friends and acquaintance all over the Union, so many as *ten* married ladies born in this century and country, who are perfectly sound, healthy, and vigorous. Not that I believe there are not more than this among the friends with whom I have associated, but among all whom I can bring to mind of whose health I have any accurate knowledge, I can not find this number of entirely sound and healthy women.

Another thing has greatly added to the impression of my own observations, and that is the manner in which my inquiries have been met. In a majority of cases, when I have asked for the number of perfectly healthy women in a given place, the first impulsive answer has been " not one." In other cases, when the reply has been more favorable, and I have asked for specifics, the result has always been such as

I

to diminish the number calculated, rather than to increase it. With a few exceptions the persons I have asked, who had not directed their thoughts to the subject, and took a favorable view of it, have expressed surprise at the painful result obtained in their own immediate circle.

But the thing which has pained and surprised me the most is the result of inquiries among the country-towns and industrial classes in our country. I had supposed that there would be a great contrast between the statements gained from persons from such places, and those furnished from the wealthy circles, and especially from cities. But such has not been the case. It will be seen that the larger portion of the accounts inserted in the preceding pages are from country-towns, while a large portion of the worst accounts were taken from the industrial classes.

As another index of the state of health among the industrial classes may be mentioned these facts: During the past year I made my usual inquiry of the wife of a Methodist clergyman, who resided in a small country-town in New York. Her reply was, "There are no healthy women where I live, and my husband says he would travel a great many miles for the pleasure of finding one."

In another case I conversed with a Baptist clergyman and his wife, in Ohio, and their united testimony gave this result in three places where his parishioners were chiefly of the industrial class. They selected at random ten families best known in each place:

Worcester, Ohio. Women in perfect health, two. In medium health, one. *Invalids, seven.*

Norwalk, Ohio. Women perfectly healthy, one, but doubtfully so. Medium, none. *Invalids, nine.*

Cleveland, Ohio. Women in perfect health, one. Medium health, two. *Invalids, seven.*

In traveling at the West the past winter, I repeatedly conversed with drivers and others among the laboring class on this subject, and always heard such remarks as these: "Well! it is strange how sickly the women are getting!" "Our women-folks don't have such health as they used to do!"

One case was very striking. An old lady from New England told me her mother had twelve children; eleven grew up healthy, and raised families. Her father's mother had fifteen children, and raised them all; and all but one, who was drowned, lived to a good old age. This lady stated that she could not remember that there was a single "weakly woman" in the town where she lived when she was young.

This lady had two daughters with her, both either delicate or diseased, and a sick niece from that same town, once so healthy when the old lady was young. This niece told me she could not think of even one really robust, strong, and perfectly healthy woman in that place! The husband of this old lady told me that in his youth he also did not know of any sickly women in the place where he was reared.

A similar account was given me by two ladies, residents of Goshen, Litchfield Co., Connecticut.

The elder lady gave the following account of her married acquaintance some forty years ago in that place:

> Mrs. L. strong and perfectly healthy. Mrs. A. healthy and strong as a horse. Mrs. N. perfectly well always. Mrs. H. strong and well. Mrs. B. strong and generally healthy, but sometimes ailing a little. Mrs. R. always well. Mrs. W. strong and well. Mrs. G. strong and hearty. Mrs. H. strong and healthy. Mrs. L. strong and healthy.

All the above persons performed their own family work.

The following account was given by the daughter of the lady mentioned above, and the list is chiefly made up of daughters of the above healthy women living at this time in the same town:

> Mrs. C. constitution broken by pelvic disorders. Mrs. P. very delicate. Mrs. L. delicate and feeble. Mrs. R. feeble and nervous. Mrs. S. bad scrofulous humors. Mrs. D. very feeble, head disordered. Mrs. R. delicate and sickly. Mrs. G. healthy. Mrs. D. healthy. Mrs. W. well.

These last three were the only healthy married women she knew in the place.

I have received statements from more than a hundred other places besides those recorded here. The larger portion of these were taken by others, or else by myself in such circumstances that I could not make the inquiries needed to render them reliable, and some I have lost.   The general impression made, even by these alone, would bring out very nearly the same result.   The proportion of the sick and delicate to those who were strong and well was, in the majority of cases, a melancholy story.   But among them were a few cases in which a very favorable statement was verified by close examination.   In several such cases, however, most of the healthy women proved to be either English, Irish, or Scotch.   In one case, a lady from a country-town, not far from Philadelphia, gave an account, showing eight out of ten perfectly healthy, and the other two were not very much out of health.   On inquiry, I found that this was a Quaker settlement, and most of the healthy ones were Quakers.

In one town of Massachusetts, the lady giving the information said all the ten she gave were healthy, but two.   Her associates were all women who were in easy circumstances, and did their own family work.   These two places, however, are the *only* instances I have found, where, on close inquiry, the majority was on the side of good health.

There is no doubt that there are many places like these two, of which some resident would report that a majority of their acquaintance were healthy women; but out of about two hundred towns and cities, located in most of the Free States, only two have as yet presented so favorable a case in the line of my inquiries during the year in which they have been prosecuted.

Let these considerations now be taken into account.   The generation represented in these statistics, by universal consent, is a feebler one than that which immediately preceded. Knowing the changes in habits of living, in habits of activity, and in respect to *pure air*, we properly infer that it must be so, while universal testimony corroborates the inference.

The present generation of parents, then, have given their children, so far as the mother has hereditary influence, feebler constitutions than the former generation received, so that most of our young girls have started in life with a more delicate organization than their mothers.   Add to this the sad picture given in a former letter of all the abuses of health suffered by the young during their early education, and what are the present prospects of the young women who are now entering married life?

This view of the case, in connection with some dreadful developments which will soon be indicated, proved so oppressive and exciting that it has been too painful and exhausting to attempt any investigation as to the state of health among young girls. But every where I go, mothers are constantly saying, "What shall I do? As soon as my little girl begins school she has the headache." Or this—"I sent my daughter to such a boarding-school, but had to take her away on account of her health."

The public schools of our towns and cities, where the great mass of the people are to be educated, are the special subject of remark and complaint in this respect.

Consider also that "man that is born of a woman" depends on her not only for the constitutional stamina with which he starts in life, but for all he receives during the developments of infancy and the training of childhood, and what are we to infer of the condition and prospects of the other sex now in the period of education?

LETTER NINETEENTH.

SOME of the results of experience and observation to be set forth in this letter, are of a description the most difficult of all possible to be brought before the public; and yet, when they are fully comprehended, it is certain that every benevolent and intelligent person must say, that nothing but the most selfish timidity would prompt to any other course.

A few preliminary words on the subject of delicacy and propriety will not be inappropriate. In regard to this, all persons agree that there are such qualities as genuine, pure, and proper modesty and delicacy, and that above almost any other virtues, these are desirable in a woman. There is no less unanimity as to the existence of a mawkish, false, and ridiculous excess, which goes by the name of prudery, false delicacy, mock modesty, and the like. Now, is there any reliable rule for our guidance in discriminating between the true and the false?

No doubt there is, and it is this: There are certain objects which are to be excluded from sight and from pictures, and there are certain topics which are to be entirely shut out from ordinary conversation. All persons, in all ages, agree as to what these objects and subjects are. And the progress of nations, both in civilization and moral worth, are distinctly shown by their less or greater strictness in these respects.

But there is a second rule not less stringent, and that is: when it is necessary in order to save from sickness, suffering, and death, or from moral contamination, to speak on these subjects, it should not only be done as fully as the case demands, but done with such an unembarrassed and full conviction of purity and rectitude, as makes it as easy and natural as it is to speak on ordinary topics.

With these rules for our guidance, the American people deserve to be placed higher than any other nation, as it regards obedience to the laws of true delicacy and refinement. Some of those topics referred to, are, even in the highest circles in England, introduced at times when there is not the least necessity for such freedoms. In France the latitude allowed is still greater, and it will be found that just in proportion as a country rises in civilization, in general culture, and *in respect for, and obedience to the Bible,* do these rules become more and more respected. The reverse is equally true, till in our downward progress we come to savages, who have almost no rules of delicacy or refinement.

But still, the American people have erred in not fully applying the second rule of propriety on these subjects. Their strictness in regard to the first has not been excessive, but their *want of discrimination in applying the second,* has led to much suffering, sickness, and death, and what is worse, to moral contamination. It is under the guidance of these rules that this letter has been written and should be read.

During the latter periods of my investigations in regard to health, I became aware, not only of the general decay of the health of my own sex, but of the terrible suffering, both physical and mental, produced by internal organic displacements, resulting chiefly from a general debility of constitution, and various abuses already indicated. And what seemed the more shocking, was the fact that so many patients of this class were young girls.

But when the fact was ascertained that, in multitudes of cases, there was no possible remedy for this appaling evil but such *daily mechanical operations, both external and internal,* as are indicated in an article from a medical writer on another page, and that this was in most cases performed with bolted doors and curtained windows, and with no one present but patient and operator, there was a painful apprehension of evils which foreshadowed future revelations. Finally, by a most remarkable combination of circumstances, developments were made and, without any prosecuting of the matter by me, facts were presented from various quarters of a most astounding nature. But before indicating these facts, some farther incidental experience should be detailed that would render what will be stated less improbable.

In my travels I have met persons of both sexes, of the highest cultivation and refinement, whose conduct was every way reputable, and whose morals were never in any way impeached, who freely advocated the doctrine that there was no true marriage but the union of persons who were in love; that such union needed not legal or religious rites, and that it was those only who were held together by such restraints, who, having ceased to love each other, were guilty of adultery in the only proper sense of the word. I have seen books and papers freely circulated that advocate the same view by the most plausible arguments.

Then, again, there are articles on physiology circulated freely, that maintain that the exercise of all the functions of body and mind is *necessary to health*, and that no perfectly-developed man or woman is possible, so long as any of the functions and propensities are held in habitual constraint. With these creeds is usually combined an entire want of reverence for the Bible as *authoritative* in teaching truth or regulating morals.

Let us now suppose the case of a physician, neither better nor worse than the majority of that honorable profession. He has read the writings of the semi-infidel school, till he has lost all reverence for the Bible as *authoritative* in faith or practice. Of course he has no guide left but his own feelings and notions. Then he gradually adopts the above views in physiology and social life, and really believes them to be founded on the *nature of things*, and the intuitive teachings of his own mind. Next he has patients of interesting person and character put under his care, and he very naturally takes the means, which these books and papers in his reach afford, to lead them to adopt *his views of truth and right* on these subjects. Then he daily has all the opportunities indicated. Does any one need more than to hear these facts to know what the not unfrequent results must be?

I will now state, in the first place, that in *no single instance* did I ever know any wrong transpire in any one of the institutions for health in which I have resided, *during the time of my residence there.* Though I had often heard suggestions and intimations, yet never, by the strictest scrutiny, could I ever learn that there was any just ground for want of entire confidence in the professional honor of any one of the medical gentlemen in whose institutions I have resided. At the same time, all the ladies with whom I conversed were unanimous in the same opinion. For, of course, a contrary opinion would immediately banish every respectable person who held it.

In regard to the health establishments implicated, only one of them was *a Water Cure*, and that one has come to an end. So that every institution now known to me of this description is, so far as I know, free from any such imputation.

These things being premised, I would state that, *during the last two years*, facts have been brought to my knowledge of a most shocking nature, and from the most unimpeachable sources. The information relied on was not received at second hand, but from ladies of the highest character and position, and involved narratives of their own hazards and escapes.

In other cases, most mournful histories were given from direct and reliable quarters of the most terrible wrongs perpetrated without any possibility of redress, except by a publicity that would inflict heavier penalties on the victims than on the wrong-doers.

So numerous were the instances that came to my knowledge *unsought*, and from so many different and unsuspected directions, and these cases involved so many guilty perpetrators, not only of those connected with health establishments but in private practice, that a most difficult and painful responsibility became apparent.

After extensive consultation as to what should be done, it has been decided that these intimations and an article from a medical source prepared for the purpose, would furnish sufficient warning without any details.

A terrific feature of these developments has been the *entire helplessness* of my sex, amidst present customs and feelings, as to any *redress* for such wrongs, and the reckless and conscious impunity felt by the wrong-doers on this account. What can a refined, delicate, sensitive woman do when thus insulted? The dreadful fear of *publicity* shuts her lips and restrains every friend. And it would seem, from some of the cases here indicated, as if it was the certainty of this that withdrew restraint, so that the very highest, not only in character but in position, have not escaped. When *such as these* have been thus assailed, who can hope to be safe?

Another alarming circumstance has been the character of several of the physicians implicated. After intimate acquaintance with some of them, I was impressed with the belief that they were, at least, men of benevolence and professional honor, while in some cases their conversation and deportment led to the hope that they were persons of consistent piety. Of course the painful inquiry has arisen, how can a woman *ever know* to whom she may safely intrust herself or her child in such painful and peculiar circumstances? No doubt the medical profession embraces multitudes of persons of the highest delicacy, honor, and principle, and those who are in long and close proximity can be sure of their rectitude. But how can *the public* discriminate? Some of these guilty men were receiving patients sent to their care by the *regular* physicians, while the great body of their patients, who had escaped all knowledge of their guilt, were earnest in their representations of their high character.

Another painful consideration is the number of cases, the short space of time in which these developments have been made, the fact that they came, as it were, by accident, and that they were met in so many different quarters; these things of course produce a strong apprehension that the extent of the evil is not by any means confined to the cases thus disclosed.

One ground of the special responsibility that has seemed to rest upon me, in reference to this painful subject, is the deep conviction acquired, not only of the extent and terrible nature of the evils resulting from a general decay and debility of the female constitution in this country, but of the *practicability of a remedy*, and of the place which *properly-conducted health establishments* must have in securing it.

During my residences at health establishments, all the books relating to the mode of medical treatment adopted were diligently studied, the views of the attending physicians were sought, and, so far as opportunities occurred, the symptoms and progress of a great variety of patients were watched, and the future result after the treatment was ended was sought by me. Comparisons were made and discussed by the physicians and myself in reference to the various methods of practice adopted, with an earnest wish on my part to form opinions from the widest possible inductions.

During my extensive journeys and residence in families in various States and sections, it has been my good fortune to be brought into frequent communion with some of the noblest and most cultivated persons, who were members of the medical profession, and who have freely given me their views on all subjects when I sought them. I have thus been enabled to look into the medical world under the most favorable influences.

The result has been two-fold: In the first place, a great respect for the profession as including a large amount of talent, cultivation, noble feelings, and high moral principle. In the next place, a conviction that the present is a period of fermentation, transition, and uncertainty, such as has never before existed; such as finds its counterpart, perhaps, only in the theological world. It would seem as if all the principles and facts of past experience were in a state of effervescence preparatory to new and more beneficent crystallizations.

In the mean time, the most intelligent, learned, and liberal seem to be cultivating a spirit of candor and patience in regard to developments that may in any way contribute to hasten the coming result of a hoped-for higher development.

In reference to what is here offered in regard to *health establishments*, the hope is indulged that it may have some influence in directing the attention of the medical world more definitely to some new efforts in this direction. The excesses and abuses that attend every new development always furnish occasion for distrust and prejudice. And yet, every enlightened and candid mind concedes that there is nothing, however wise and good, that is not liable to be thus marred in one way or another.

The regular physician, when he prescribes simple diet, air, exercise, and relief from care, finds that he can not enforce his prescriptions on those who are encompassed with all the business and customs of life.   To meet this difficulty why can not institutions of the kind indicated in this work be brought into operation by the powerful influence and patronage of the regular and associated medical profession?   And why should not all improvements and discoveries that may have been made, even, it may be, by charlatans, be examined and secured by those who hold the highest position in public confidence, and who claim to seek the accumulated wisdom of all ages and of all experimenters?

There are processes which can restore a distorted form to symmetry, which can remedy the most extreme internal displacements, and which can cure the most terrible of all diseases.   These methods I have never seen or known to be adopted, except in health establishments.   Indeed, it is almost impossible to prosecute them in any other circumstances.

And yet, the discovery and practice of these methods has been attended with great abuses, not only in the establishments where they originated, but in private practice also.

It is in reference to these and other dangers, as well as to direct attention to the true methods of relief, that a medical article has been furnished which should now be read. It will be found as Note I., with this heading:

COMMUNICATION FROM MRS. DR. R. B. GLEASON.

PART FIFTH.

LETTER TWENTIETH.

THE concluding portion of this work is devoted to the *remedies* to be sought for the evils set forth.

It has been the conviction that there *are* remedies—that these remedies are practicable, and that, when the evils and the remedies are fairly understood, they will be adopted by the American people, which has sustained courage and hope under the heavy pressure which such views and facts as have been presented would naturally produce.

But inasmuch as *a resort to health establishments* will be suggested as an important measure in many cases, some preliminary remarks on this topic will be introduced.

Most of these institutions, and certainly the best ones, are what are called *Water Cures*. Before proceeding it may be desirable to give a short statement of the *philosophy* of the Water Cure.

Cold water taken internally operates first to dissolve and thin the morbid accumulations in all parts of the system, and thus prepare them for ejection through the skin, lungs, kidneys, and bowels. Next it tends to equalize the circulation by thinning and removing these morbid obstructions, so that the blood can flow equally in every part. Next it stimulates the capillaries to quicker action all over the body. Water taken into the stomach is drawn into the circulation in ten or fifteen minutes, and as the great mass of the blood courses through the body six or eight times every hour, it is seen that the water in that time may visit nearly every part. If more is taken than the body needs, the kidneys draw it off and send it out. Cold water is a *tonic;* that is, it operates to give stronger action to the minute capillaries, and this, like the exercise of the muscles, gives increase of vigor. Thus, cold water taken internally operates to purify the blood, to equalize the circulation, and to strengthen the capillary action by increased exercise.

Cold water applied *externally*, in baths, operates in several ways. In the first place, it is a tonic to the nerves and capillaries of the skin. And as there is more nerve matter and more blood in the skin than in all the other capillaries of the body, there is no mode of applying tonic remedies so potent and so readily within reach.

Next, cold water can be applied in *local baths* to draw the blood from one portion of the body where there is an excess, to another part where there is a deficiency and consequent debility. The sitz and foot baths are of this nature. If we need blood and increased action in any particular part, *cold* is applied by water. The capillaries contract and send their blood inward, reporting to the brain the need of the part. Instantly there is a return of a greater supply than before. This process can be continued till a habit is induced, and thus the part is strengthened.

Next, cold water, in drawing off heat from the body, and quickening the action of the capillaries, hastens the process of *change* which is going on all over the system in sending off old, decayed matter, and replacing it with new material furnished by the lungs and stomach. It is thus that the Water Cure quickens the appetite to supply the increased demand.

Lastly, cold water can be applied as a kind of *poultice to the skin*. In this case, the *moisture* and *warmth* draw the blood to the capillaries of the skin, and at the same time stimulate the lymphatic absorbents to quicker action. By this method morbid humors are drawn from the internal organs to the skin, and thence are thrown off. The wet sheet is a cold-water poultice for the whole body. The wet bandages, worn over diseased parts, are smaller poultices. Both act to draw blood from within to the skin, and then to abstract from it the morbid humors.

When we consider that the surface of skin comprises fifteen square feet, that this surface is made up of millions of perspiration tubes, oil-secreting glands, and sensitive, nervous reticulations, it can be seen that we have the means of influencing the brain and nerves, and, indeed, the whole system, as can be done in no other way. We can depress one part, and stimulate another; bring the blood to the surface, drive it inward, equalize and cleanse it, and apply a universal tonic to its whole net-work of nerves by means of this one simple, pure, and universal element.

But the medical and scientific application of cold water for the cure of disease is only one of the benefits to be obtained in these health establishments. The great thing secured is a rational, intelligent commencement of *obedience to the laws of health*. As the body is, by the use of cold water, dissolved and carried off by quickened action, so it is built up with pure and healthful materials by a simple diet. Tea, coffee, alcoholic drinks, opium, tobacco, spices, and condiments of all sorts are relinquished. Fruits, vegetables, broths, one kind of meat, coarse bread, and a great variety of simples, such as cracked wheat, hominy, and the like, are provided, and the patient must eat these or starve, or go somewhere else for food.

Next, and chief, after every bath the patient is required to bring on a glow by exercise in the open air, and as baths are taken four and five times a day, this secures a considerable amount of pure air for the lungs, as well as exercise for the lower limbs. In addition to this, several Water Cures have adopted a system of calisthenics that exercises all the other muscles of the body.

Besides this, the patients are withdrawn from all their business and cares. The brain has a chance to rest; while the baths and walking furnish occupation that is cheered by the stimulus of hope. At the same time, in these gatherings, every person finds one or more sympathizing associates in walks and sports, and thus time never seems to hang heavily.

In a few institutions, also, such arrangements for *ventilation* are *enforced* as secures to the patients *pure air* both by night and by day.

Finally, by means of the books treating on health and the Water Cure, which abound at such places, by means of lectures from the physicians, and by the discussions on these topics among the patients themselves, there comes to be an intelligent conviction of the reality and obligations of the laws of health, which is carried to multitudes of homes to modify and improve the habits of a household. At the same time, the various simple articles of diet, and healthful modes of cooking are learned, and transferred to home-circles.

But while these inestimable benefits are secured, it is no less true that, as in all things human, some evils are involved, and, as being forewarned is being forearmed, these should also be pointed out.

Among the first is the great want of care in the larger portion of these establishments to secure an adequate supply of *pure air*. In a place where multitudes of patients congregate, whose morbid humors are being drawn off through the skin, surely extraordinary means should be used to ventilate every room and passage both by night and by day; while all those articles which are filled with these excretions should daily be purified by fresh air, and at such a distance from the premises as not to interfere with the purity of the atmosphere around it. In this matter there is great room for improvement. In many of these institutions very little notice is taken of the state of the atmosphere through the house, especially in the small and close-packed lodging-rooms, which eight hours out of twenty-four furnish all the supplies for the lungs of their inmates. Such establishments need to have an official, whose express duty it shall be to provide pure air; and all needful expense should be given to secure it as much as to secure the water used. For, of the two, the pure air is of the most vital importance. Had this matter been properly cared for, it is probable that double the amount of good would have been secured.

Another very great deficiency in the larger portion of these institutions, in time past, has been that there has been no method for securing to the patients the *appropriate* exercise of all the muscles of the body, such as alone can secure equable and full physical development. In most cases, all the exercise required has been a walk after the baths, while the muscles of the arms and trunk have been entirely neglected. In two or three cases, where the attending physician seemed to have more just views on the subject, he not only *prescribed* the kind and amount of exercise to be taken, but was present himself, at regular seasons, to see that his prescriptions were obeyed; and any failure was dealt with as common physicians deal with patients who neglect the *doses* prescribed. It was in such cases that the most marked results of improvement or cure have been observed.

Another defect in many institutions is that want of systematic instruction on the laws of health and the philosophy of the treatment adopted, which alone can secure a hearty, intelligent, and cheerful co-operation of the patient and physician. In those Cures where the physician has adopted this plan, many very valuable results are secured. One of the best is, that on leaving the establishment, many evils are escaped, and continued health or improvement secured by the influence of this instruction. And all the families of patients, so instructed, also reap incalculable benefits.

Another defect in many of these institutions is the want of proper arrangements for the preservation of personal modesty while taking the treatment. In many cases the curtains that should protect the plunge, sitz, and half baths, are entirely wanting, while in others, they are allowed to to be unused by any who are unrefined enough to choose it. This is not only in bad taste, but its tendency is deteriorating. The cultivation of personal modesty in childhood is of the greatest importance to future delicacy and purity of character, and all arrangements which tend to destroy it should be earnestly reprobated. A truly modest and refined person is one who, where a thing is necessary or inevitable, always submits with the most quietness. And it is owing to this fact that very many are silent in their disapprobation of what they suppose to be irremediable, when their protest *might* produce a remedy, and save others from the same evil and discomfort. If every one, hereafter, who disapproves this custom, would calmly and decidedly oppose it, and use all their influence to secure a remedy, the evil would soon be ended. And if it is not remedied, its evil tendencies will be developed in ways that have already become apparent, but which, at present, need not be indicated.

Another great evil involved in the management of these institutions, has been the *excesses* in treatment. These have

K

resulted, in the first place, from the fact that the system originated among the hardy, phlegmatic German race, and needed modifications to adapt it to the excitable, sensitive, and worn-out constitutions of the American people, that could only be discovered by experiment. During the ten years of its trial in this country it has constantly gained in successful results, and almost as constantly diminished in the energy of its application. In two or three cases I observed its power appeared very much diminished by too great amelioration, and probably the happy medium has been obtained in most of the institutions now patronized.

The excesses referred to relate to *exercise* as well as to the application of water. Every human body has its reservoir of nervous energy, some large, and some very small, with all grades between. The amount of this resource is regulated by original constitution, by the wear and tear and exhaustion of life, and by disease and its attending circumstances. Now the grand difficulty in the management both of water and exercise, as remedial, is that both physicians and patients are insidiously led on by the feeling that "more produces more," without any need of careful and scientific limitations.

There is nothing that requires more careful watching and good judgment, than to adapt the amount of water-treatment and exercise to the degree of nervous resource which each patient may possess. And, probably, more than half the benefits of both methods have been lost by such excesses that the nervous fountain had only enough of supply for the excessive tax put upon it by the treatment, and had little to spare for the struggle that otherwise would have thrown off the disease. This evil comes sometimes in spite of the care and caution of the physician, but more frequently for the want of it. The fact that the chief difficulty is to bring patients to exercise enough, leads to measures and motives that stimulate a certain class that need rather to be held back. At the same time, there arises a spirit of emulation, and a pride, and self-gratulation at achievements which strongly tempt to excess.

Another great defect in many such establishments, is the want of *intelligent* supervision in the nursing department

All that the physician can ordinarily do, is to prescribe the treatment and watch the results. He can not oversee and watch the nurses and patients to see that his directions are properly obeyed. But this department should be attended to by some well-educated person, who understands the nature of the treatment, and has authority to supervise the nurses.

In most cases the drudgery of the nursing department is executed by ignorant, heedless, and inexperienced persons, who know nothing of the processes which they are carrying forward. And yet they temper the water for baths, and are expected to see that all the directions of the physician are properly executed. But such persons can not properly be trusted without intelligent supervision. There have been multitudes of cases, known to me personally, of serious and lasting injuries inflicted from this cause. New patients can not be relied on to take care of themselves. Young and thoughtless patients need a person who has *official* authority to enforce their obedience to the physician's prescriptions.

Moreover, the care of the sheets and bandages that should daily be scalded, and the sweating apparatus that should daily be taken out of the premises and aired properly, can never safely be trusted to a class of unintelligent, irresponsible menials, without any supervision. No intelligent person who has watched this department of the Water Cure treatment, can fail to have felt that there is a serious evil to to be remedied here.

Another defect in several such institutions is the want of an intelligent, refined, and sympathizing matron to fulfill the offices of a mother in the care and superintendence of the whole concern. A person possessing these traits in such a position, can do almost as much as nurse and physician united in promoting that *state of mind* in patients most favorable of all others to health. None but those who have felt the contrast between the institutions so provided and those that are destitute, can understand the value and importance of this arrangement.

Another deficiency in some of these establishments is the want of that moral and religious influence, which is especially needed by large communities so diverse in their notions and habits, and yet so closely affiliated as to involve great liabilities to evil influences. The assembling of the whole family every morning to hear the Scriptures read, to unite in devotional singing, and to join in supplications for the Divine Wisdom to guide and Divine Power to bless the object for which they are made one family, has a most harmonizing and healthful influence.

Then when the physicians are men of true benevolence and piety, the most favorable of all opportunities are presented not only for the healing of the body but to minister to the mind diseased. Such can and will watch very narrowly that, in such susceptible seasons, none but the most healthful and invigorating moral atmosphere shall surround the objects of sympathy and care. Such physicians can detect who are tempters and who are the weak and unguarded, and watch them as a shepherd guards his fold. Oh, thrice blessed are they who, in this relation and in these offices, can so closely imitate the Great Shepherd and Physician of souls.

As a matter of course, my frequent visits to Health Establishments has resulted from the *success* that has attended the methods pursued, a success altogether beyond any thing I have ever known from any other attempts to remedy *chronic* complaints. I could fill pages with accounts of interesting cases of those who had tried all methods of medication in vain.

As a specimen, I have seen one young girl, who was refused at first by the physician as an incurable consumptive, transformed, by eight months' treatment, from a thin, pale, delicate creature that seemed just ready for the grave to a strong, fat, red-cheeked, healthy woman, as different from her former self as light from darkness.

I have seen the dyspeptic, whom physicians and friends had given over as incurable, with nothing more to do but die, changed to an elastic, sprightly woman, with as much health and capacity in her new duties as wife and mother as American women ordinarily enjoy.

I have seen approaching blindness and deafness entirely remedied; neuralgia, with its thousand agonies, conquered;

a great variety of skin complaints and bad humors cured, and multitudes of internal organic disorders and displacements remedied. In short, I have seen almost "every ill that flesh is heir to," in one institution or another, yielding to the methods here indicated.

And it should be remembered that this strong conviction has been induced by observing results in very imperfectly conducted institutions, and during the period of *experimenting* on a new method of practice. Still more should it be remembered that this impression has been gained in communities of invalids with chronic complaints, who had been poisoned by medicines and worn down by all sorts of previous abuse and mismanagement. This treatment demands so much time and is so very expensive, that few will resort to it till all other methods are tried and all hope of other remedy abandoned.

And yet I have seen many cases that could not be cured, and some that from one cause or another were more injured than benefited. But the cases where I have known most of the injuries to result, were under the hands of incautious or inexperienced practitioners, at the early period of water treatment, when the "heroic" method was being tested. And the impression, so common at that time, that "a crisis" must be induced, and that any increase of bad symptoms was a harbinger of this desired result, often deluded both patient and physician to *continue* injurious methods even after the evil results were manifest.

This dangerous liability is remedied by the practice of intermitting the treatment when bad symptoms increase. For if a crisis is approaching this is the best method to accelerate it, while if it is not soon developed, then it is clear that the treatment is not the right one, and a change is made.

The great advantage of the Water Cure is, that the process is so *slow* that no great harm can be *suddenly* effected, while the indications of mistaken treatment can be obeyed before any evil is done.

The fact that these institutions have been conducted by some of the most conservative of the *regular* Allopathic school, and that they are patronized and recommended by physicians of *all* schools, is a substantial proof of their high claims to confidence.

The general result of all my observations at Water Cures has been the earnest wish and prayer that such institutions, with all these improved methods, may be multiplied all over the land, as the safest and surest methods of relieving debilitated constitutions and curing chronic ailments. And I believe no philanthropist, who has funds to invest for the relief of human suffering, could do a greater service to humanity, than by providing health institutions of this class for the *gratuitous* or *cheap* treatment of *the poor*. Thousands of such, all over the land, are lying in hopeless suffering, a burden to their poor families, and suffering untold agonies of body and mind, that by such benefactions would be relieved.

LETTER TWENTY-FIRST.

SUBSTITUTES FOR FAMILY MEDICINES.

It is probable that there has been no more fruitful cause of disease and suffering among the American people than the use of family and quack medicines, unguided by medical science and skill.

To appreciate this, we need to refer to the fact set forth in the letter on *abuses of the stomach*, that the excesses in quantity, and the wrong selections of food, keep the blood and the whole system in an overloaded state. This being so, the true remedy for the greater portion of temporary ailments for which medicines are taken, would be to stop pouring into the stomach, and give nature time and strength to dispose of this excess. A fast of one, two, or three days will remedy multitudes of sicknesses; as thus all the over-tasked functions of the body can rest, and the excreting organs throw off the excess.

Instead of this, some medicine is thrown into the stomach which is of the nature of a poison. The whole organism is instantly aroused to resist the intruder. The brain sends its nervous mandates to every part to summon aid. The blood hastens to the stomach and intestines, in order to pour through them the slimy mucus that speedily encases the mischief maker, and thus it is carried off through the lower intestines. At the same time, this operation destroys all appetite. Thus the blood is relieved of some of its excess by the emptying out of the mucous secretions, and the stomach is kept from receiving food for a day or two. This being done, the patient feels better, and the poison that made all this commotion is called the cure.

But such an operation as this never takes place without a drain on the constitutional energies, while in many cases some portion of the poison thus thrown into the stomach is absorbed by the blood, and being carried through the body, lodges here and there in its minute and delicate tissues. This is especially the case with the metallic medicines, which being heavier, are not so easily carried off. I have again and again seen, at Water Cures, the bandages worn by patients over diseased parts by one week's use turn yellow, green, and brown, and become rotten in texture, by the passing off of poisonous substances thus lodged in the skin.

In one case, a lady whose spine for years had been subjected to medical applications, was visited by me daily to observe a result of this nature. She took every Monday a towel that was whole and pinned it around her waist as a wet bandage, so that it would bring the same part every day over her spine. And three successive weeks those towels, which I saw whole and good at the beginning of the week, at its close I found marked with brown and yellow spots, through which I could pass my fingers as if they had been scorched brown with fire.

And in multitudes of cases I have seen the sweating sheets and bandages stained with red, green, yellow, or brown, and in some cases could distinctly perceive the peculiar smell of certain medicines that had been taken freely. All physicians and nurses at Water Cures will testify to the same facts.

Most of the popular quack medicines, advertised as cures for almost every disease, contain either calomel or quinine, or strong metallic or other poisons, that stimulate the brain or drain the blood in the way above stated. Most of them, at the same time, tend to induce costiveness by debilitating the intestinal canal. Many of them induce a tendency of blood to those parts, producing inflammations, piles, and other distressing complaints.

Every thing taken into the stomach is either food and drink that nourish the body, or it is inert, unassimilating matter that simply passes off, or it is what is more or less of the nature of poison which, whether as stimulant or sedative, produces unnatural and therefore unhealthful action of all the parts influenced. Tonics tend to destroy tone, cathartics tend to produce constipation, emetics tend to de-

bilitate stomach, liver, and bowels, while such medicines as
mercury, arsenic, antimony, iodine, and the like, are insidious poisons that establish themselves in the delicate tissues
of the body, debilitating the constitution, and generating
innumerable evils. It is the wise and skillful physician
alone who can use these agents properly, if they ever are
needed.

The poisons that have probably done the most mischief
are *calomel* and *quinine*. These are what are deemed the
grand remedies for the chief diseases of our newer States,
resulting from the climate, habits of diet, and the malaria
of decayed vegetable matter in fresh soil.

Bilious complaints usually result from excess in eating
and a diet unsuited to a warm climate. Carbonaceous food,
such as oils, butter, pork, sugar, and molasses, all tend to
fill the blood with an excess of carbon. It is the office of
the liver to draw off this excess. It is overtaxed, and then
ceases its work. Mercury, or calomel, has the power of
stimulating this organ. So instead of taking less food into
the stomach, and selecting that which has least carbon, a
dose of calomel is taken. This stimulates the liver to unnatural action, and it is roused from its attempt to rest and
forced to double duty. Then "a cathartic" is taken to
"clear out the calomel." This is some kind of poison
which summons the blood from all points to the intestines,
to deposit the needed mucus to envelop and carry it off.
Thus the system is for a time relieved of its excess. But
every time this is done the constitution is undermined, till
finally a chronic weakness settles on the liver, stomach, or
bowels. Meantime appetite fails, and the system, not so
greatly taxed by food, accommodates to the weakened organs, and a sort of dying half life is the result.

In the case of chills and fever, the inhaled malaria of a
bad atmosphere poisons the whole organism, and at periodic
turns there is a grand effort of nature to shake it off. Quinine is a medicine that acts as a quiet, unperceived stimulant to the brain and nervous system. This being put into
the stomach, acts on the brain and nerves, and gives them
temporary strength, and for a time the enemy retires. In a
good constitution it is sometimes the case that there is no

great harm done, and the person is thus made well. But the repetition of this method often undermines the nervous system fatally. I have friends who, from the frequent use of quinine, have brought on deafness, vertigo, heart disease, and many nervous evils that will probably follow them through life.

In cases where biliary, stomach, and other intestinal affections are brought on by care, anxiety, or any overworking of the brain, simple diet, rest, sleep, and a great deal of exercise in the open air are better than any medicines. When these affections are caused by excess of food or by the wrong selection, the evil can be *starved out*. Three or four days of fasting will do it far safer than calomel or any medicine.

There are some of the processes of the Water Cure which all intelligent and candid physicians will say are perfectly safe, that if adopted in families in place of pills and other doses, would save from much evil. After these processes have been fairly tried, few would ever wish to return to medicines as a remedy for these most common ailments. They have been furnished by some of the most experienced physicians in the water treatment.

TREATMENT FOR BILIOUSNESS.

A pack in the wet sheet at 11 A.M. for three quarters of an hour, to be followed with a washing of the whole body in water at 72. Keep the head cool with a wet cloth.

At 4 P.M. take a hot bath (either sitz or full bath) at 110 to 120, followed by a wash in cool water at 80. Keep the head cool. [Hot fomentations over the liver are often very useful.] Drink from four to six tumblers of cold water before breakfast. If the stomach is too irritable for this, drink warm crust coffee. Wear a wet bandage around the body over the liver, covered with a dry double bandage, and exercise in the open air, but not to great fatigue.

TREATMENT FOR CHILLS AND FEVER.

In cases where chills and fever occur, this method of using water will be found effective.

In the *fever*, pack in the wet sheet from ten to thirty

minutes. Use water at 72 to wet the sheet. Wash off in water at 80. If nauseated, use warm water as a vomit.

In the *chill*, take a hot sitting bath with feet in hot water from one half to three quarters of an hour, keeping the head cool with a wet cloth on the head.

If the fever is high, repeat the packing every half hour till it is reduced. No danger at all in this. Wash off in cool water, and rub well. Exercise in the open air, but not to fatigue. Sit and sleep in a cool and well-ventilated room, and keep on enough clothing to prevent chilliness.

In most families the medicine chest is most frequently visited in cases of colds, constipation, or diarrhea. These methods are far safer and better than medicine.

TREATMENT FOR A COLD IN THE HEAD.

On going to bed, cover the head, face, and neck with a wet towel, leaving just opening enough to breathe freely around the mouth and nose. Cover this with a small woolen blanket so as to keep the head and neck warm. Keep up a gentle perspiration during the whole night. In the morning wash the head, face, and neck with cold water, dry the hair, or keep the head from cold till it is dry.

If too much trouble is made by wetting the hair, treat the face and neck thus.

TREATMENT FOR A COLD ON THE LUNGS.

Pack in a sheet wet in water at 80 for three quarters of an hour at 11 A.M. Wash off in water at 70.

At night, just before going to bed, take a hot sitting bath, with feet also in hot water at 110, for fifteen minutes. Wash off in water at 70. Wear a wet bandage over the chest all night, and keep up a gentle perspiration. Hot fomentations of the chest on retiring are very efficacious.

The *certain* cure of a cold in the head or on the lungs depends on treating it *immediately*. If it is allowed to run on a day or two, the above treatment will palliate and shorten the evil, but, if taken at the commencement, it will stop it entirely.

These methods open the closed pores and draw the blood to the skin, and thus relieve the internal organs.

TREATMENT FOR CONSTIPATION.

Eat coarse bread and cooked fruit. Drink three tumblers of water before breakfast, and two on going to bed. Exercise a great deal in pure air, and sleep in the same. Solicit nature by efforts at a regular time directly after a meal. If this does not avail, use cool water injections— half a pint at once, after breakfast and on going to bed— the last to be retained if possible.

TREATMENT FOR DIARRHEA OR DYSENTERY.

Stop eating entirely, that the irritated intestines may rest. If the stomach is not irritable, drink cold water often—a third of a tumbler at once. Take a sitting bath twice a day at 70, following it by friction of the skin. Wear a wet bandage around the abdomen, and keep from any chills by enough clothing. After every passage from the bowels take an injection of cold water at 65. Use for food gruel of coarse wheat; in dysentery, some mucilaginous drinks like gum Arabic or slippery-elm tea.

In case of fever, pack in the wet sheet half an hour, using water at 75.

Every physician will say these methods are *safe*. Try them before going to the medicine chest.

If a thermometer is wanting, "take the chill off" from the coldest water by adding, say a quart of boiling water to a pailful of very cold water, and it is about at 65, say another quart will make it 70 or so.

If these prescriptions fail, do not trust your own skill, but send for a physician.

DIRECTIONS FOR PACKING, BATHS, AND FOMENTATIONS.

For Packing. Spread on a bed, first, a thick cotton comforter; over that a woolen blanket, and over that a piece of linen sheet which is only long enough to reach from neck to ankles, and which is wrung out in cool water. Wrap the patient first in the sheet, not putting it on the feet, and then draw the blanket and tuck it closely all around, especially about the neck, to keep out the air. Then do the same with the comforter. If the room is cold, spread on another comforter. This process, if repeated, will always reduce *any* fever for the time, even if it can not remove the cause.

For the sitz bath. Take a wash-tub, and put in water enough to cover the hips. Wear a warm, loose garment, and, if cold, a blanket over. Rub the parts immersed.

For a foot bath. The water in this bath should not come quite up to the ankle-bone, and the feet should be constantly rubbed together. It often relieves a headache, if protracted for half or three quarters of an hour.

Fomentations. A wet linen compress, with dry cloth over, and a tin vessel or bottle filled with hot water, placed so as to keep the compress warm, is the easiest method. Another method is to keep water hot on the fire or stove. Dip cloths in, and wring them out by putting them in a towel and wringing that. The compress should increase in heat every time till it is as hot as can be borne.

Every use of hot water should be followed with cold, to prevent debility of the skin.

In the water treatment, in *no case* is water to be used very cold at first. A preliminary process of several days, in which the water is made a little cooler each day, is indispensable. In severe disease no person should adopt the water treatment except under the guidance of a physician who has had experience in it; for it is a very powerful agency, requiring skill and experience in such cases.

In reference to the use of medicine, every person must perceive there has been a great change among physicians. Every year there is less and less reliance placed by them on medicines thrown into the body, whose chemical and vital processes are so complicated and mysterious, while more and more resort is had to the restorative influences which nature herself provides when the laws of health are properly obeyed.

Those physicians that not only examine the pulse and tongue, but attend to diet, ventilation, and the care of the skin and insist on fresh air and abundant exercise, find that the prescriptions to the apothecary are constantly diminishing; and the public are beginning to test the skill of their medical advisers by this standard.

LETTER TWENTY-SECOND.

It is the object of this letter to present evidence that there has been such results induced by the neglect of the laws of health, by the various abuses set forth, and by other developments of the age, that *the whole of our adult population* should be apprised of certain dangers as yet but little known, and should thus be induced to institute protective customs and precautions, which at former periods were not so much demanded.

The first point for consideration is whether the period of *protection by ignorance* to the young is not hopelessly past, and to be supplanted by the *protection of knowledge*. To illustrate this, one fact of personal observation will suffice. From the age of nine till eighteen my whole youth was spent with boarding-school girls, in a place where nearly *one hundred a year* came from all parts of the land; a portion of whom, for years, boarded in my father's family. During that whole time I never heard, so far as I can recollect, an impure or indecent communication, and I was as profoundly ignorant on all those topics that are by custom excluded from common conversation, at eighteen, as I was at two years of age.

In the early part of my experience as the principal of a large boarding-school, I had an English work put into my hands containing warnings in regard to certain dangerous practices, especially at boarding-schools, which are indicated in Mrs. Gleason's article. The whole thing was perfectly unintelligible, and when I went to several of my matron friends for information, I could not find any one that had ever heard of such a thing. I then consulted my medical adviser, and was told that there was no occasion to think or do any thing on the subject. And there the matter was ended for years.

Such ignorance as this can now rarely be found, if the testimony of mothers and teachers all over the land can be relied on. On the contrary, the children at this day, to a wide extent, know far more than the parents ever learned in a former generation through their whole lives, while not unfrequently they find, with dismay and horror, their little ones losing strength and a healthful hue from a cause never feared or imagined. The only question now to be settled seems to be, who shall be the teachers of the young on such subjects, their pure, judicious, and proper guardians, or the vulgar and vile?

Mothers who have trained their sons with all the care and watchfulness possible; who imagined their minds as pure as the lilies of the garden; who had sent them to just those schools most celebrated for the greatest care, and strong moral and religious influences, have told me of books they have found in their rooms with details and descriptions that might horrify even the vicious; and they were then told that "the boys were reading them at school, and offered them to the others."

I have seen books and papers, ostensibly designed for good, and circulated freely, even by well-meaning persons, that, it seemed to me, *could not be made worse*, as it respects their insidious and unsuspected influence. And the writings that abound in all quarters, prepared with the best intentions, are often so gross, so injudicious, and so unrefined in all respects, as justly to shock and offend the delicate and pure.

In this matter, as in all others of importance, if the judicious, well-educated, and refined, do not take the control of the matter, it will fall into the hands of the uncultivated and erratic, and the people, pressed by their necessities, will follow such leaders for want of any safer ones.

Another development of the age demands especial attention. In the medical world, new and powerful agents have been discovered, that are serviceable both in dentistry and medical treatment, and yet involve great liabilities to dangerous preversions. Among these are animal magnetism and its kindred developments, the "spirit rapping" agency, whatever it may be. This is a topic which demands a larger space than can here be given, and a note at the end contains farther views that may be read at another time. But there are dangers in this direction which, until very lately, have not been properly understood, or estimated by most of my acquaintances, or by myself.

These are such as make it needful to warn every woman never to submit to any such influence unless for the relief of some great evil, and in such a case, if practicable, to secure it from one of her own sex, or at any rate in the presence of a third person.

Since many of my pupils have become matrons, I have been told by them of liabilities which perfect purity and innocence involve, which ought to be considered in regulating protecting customs for the young. They have told me, what I also had occasion to observe frequently myself, of the power which a teacher, even of the same sex, may exert on the affections and susceptibilities of pupils, so that in some cases they may become morbid and excessive. There is a period when the young, especially if highly gifted, find an outbursting of sensibilities that they have not learned to control.

At such periods, if entirely ignorant of the reasons why certain rules of decorum in expression and manners are instituted, they are liable to say and do things which, if properly construed, are the highest evidence of innocence and purity, and yet are most liable to be misconstrued and misunderstood. This is a matter which, even in a healthy and ordinary condition of the physical system, demands consideration. But especially is this necessary in reference to liabilities indicated in the last topic in Mrs. Gleason's article.

In this view of the matter, the placing of young girls in the care of teachers of the other sex, in the hands of physicians, or even under the instructions of clergymen, ought to be regulated by precautions and customs that now are rarely enforced. And especially the freedoms that have been tolerated in the associations of the young of both sexes, require new restraints and customs. There must, ere long, be painful developments in these directions that will give new force to these intimations.

The truth should be plainly set forth, that the snares, temptations, and dangers that will assail the young at this and the coming period, are altogether beyond any thing known in our past history, or any thing which is now imagined.

At the same time many restraints of circumstances and opinions have been removed. The press is teeming with dangerous and pernicious literature, like the pestilent frogs of Egypt; and there is no place so secret or retired that will long be free from the inroad. Then the style of educating the young, at once so debilitating and so stimulating, is fraught with innumerable dangers.

Then the restraints of the religious principle are failing in many directions. The laws that guard the family relation are more dependent on Christianity than any other, because here is the place where human passions always make the fiercest onset. *Without the Bible* every man sets up his own opinions and notions as the rule of right, and who is then to decide?

In the higher circles, Madame Sand, and others of that genus, with their fascinating style and false principles, combine with pretended teachers of physiology and hygiene. In the lower classes Mormonism and " Spiritualism" take the same course. Meantime thousands of insidious influences are warring against the authority of that Book, which alone claims to decide the contested questions, so important to human happiness, with the stern assumption " Thus saith the Lord." Men, in this highly-stimulating age, are not to be regulated in their outbursting passions by theories of morals educed by the genius of man and the light of reason. They must be met by the imposing and incontestible authority of an Almighty Creator, or the masses will become the slaves of their own passions and propensities.

But there is one especial cause of alarm which should command instant and earnest attention. In Mrs. Gleason's article have been indicated *certain deformities and internal displacements*, which have resulted from the *general debility*

L

of constitution, brought on both mature woman and young girls by over-excited brains, by the want of pure air, simple diet, and exercise, and by the abominations of fashionable dress.

But the *terrible sufferings* that are sometimes thus induced can never be conceived of, or at all appreciated from any use of language. Nothing that the public can be made to believe on this subject will ever equal the reality of what I, again and again, have personally known. It is not that I have so often seen, not only mature persons and mothers, but fair young girls shut up for months and years as helpless and suffering invalids from this cause. This may be found all over the land. But it is the *horrible extremity of suffering* often involved in certain forms of this evil, which no woman of feeble constitution can ever be certain may not be her doom. Not that in all cases this extremity of suffering is involved, but none can say which will escape it.

In regard to this, and in reference to cases that have come to my personal knowledge, I can truly say that, if I must choose for a friend or a child, on the one hand the horrible torments inflicted by savage Indians or cruel inquisitors on their victims, or on the other, the protracted agonies that I have seen and known to be endured as the result of such deformities and displacements, I should choose the former as a merciful exchange.

And yet this is the fate that is coming to meet the young as well as the mature in every direction. And tender parents are unconsciously leading their lovely and hapless daughters to this horrible doom.

This it is, that has pressed like lead upon my heart and burned like fire in my bones, as for more than two years of debility, anxiety, and infirmity, I have been striving to bring this subject to the attention of the American people.

There is no excitement of the imagination in what is here indicated. If the facts and details *could* be presented, they would send a groan of terror and horror all over the land. For it is not one *class*, or one *section*, that is endangered. In every part of our country the evil is progressing. There is scarcely a State in the union that has not been represented among this class of sufferers, while they have testified to similar sufferings among their friends.

And, as if these dreadful evils were not enough, there have been added methods of medical treatment at once useless, torturing to the mind, and involving great liabilities to immoralities. The warnings in Mrs. Gleason's article can not be too anxiously pondered by every parent, and especially by every woman.

At the same time, the medical profession, in view of such disclosures, can not but feel that their honor, as well as the safety of woman, demands some protective customs, which shall be stringently enforced by their decided authority. It is said that the instructors in medical schools advise their pupils always to demand the presence of some female attendant in all cases where any such liabilities exist. This advice the profession have influence sufficient to change into an imperative custom, and when this is secured a most effective remedy for this part of the evil will be provided.

LETTER TWENTY-THIRD.

WHAT IS TO BE DONE?

WE have now reached the final portion of this work, in which is to be suggested more definitely the *remedies* for the evils that have been set forth.

In pursuing this, it is clear that the undertaking is equaled in importance only by the difficulties to be overcome. To change essentially the habits, customs, and daily practices of a whole nation, in regard to exercise, ventilation, food, drink, amusements, medical treatment, and modes of training the young, certainly is a most Herculean undertaking; and yet nothing less than this will at all meet the case.

But then the American people never fail in any thing they choose to undertake, and they would feel a pride and pleasure in accomplishing a wonderful and beneficent change, and one, too, that would *in all respects set them at the head of the human race.*

For it is granted by all physiologists and naturalists that the mingling of races is the surest mode of securing the highest physical developments of the human family. The superiority of the Anglo-Saxon race is always traced to the happy combination of the British, Celtic, Saxon, and Norman races. In America a new development is to be made, by the union of almost every civilized race, and the eventual result must be the highest type of human physical development, so far as this single cause shall have its influence.

If, in addition to this, the American people could become enlightened as to the true modes of physical training both of themselves and their offspring, and should excel all nations in customs and habits conformed to the laws of health, both of body and mind, what a glorious development of humanity would ensue! And why may not this be hoped for, and undertaken as a direct and practical aim? What human undertaking ever was started that so directly appealed to the personal interest of every individual of a nation, and yet, at the same time, was so free from all antagonistic influences and combinations?

The first thing suggested then is, that appropriate means be taken to make *the whole people understand this subject*, as presented in this work. If suitable measures for this end were adopted, in a few months every man and woman in this nation who can read, might have this little book placed in their hands. The labor of simplifying and condensing a subject usually so enveloped in technics, and thus putting it in reach of the most ordinary capacity, has been what few can understand, and was done with this very end in view.

Men never can be made to obey what to them are *empirical* rules of health. They must understand the construction of their bodies, the functions of the several organs, and their modes of healthful action. They must understand the nature of the atmosphere they breathe, and of the food they eat, and the influences of their habits, customs, and employments on the various organs and functions of their bodies. When this is secured, reason, conscience, self-love, domestic affection, and religion, furnish motives of obedience to laws perceived to be wise and necessary, and whose penalties are inevitable.

They also must have clear and practical ideas of the exact course each one individually should pursue, in remedying the evils here presented. In reference to this, more exact and minute details will now be set forth, under the main topics.

PURE AIR AND VENTILATION.

This topic takes the lead of all others in importance and difficulty. The fact that the Greeks lived most of the year out-doors, and that in their houses they never breathed any but pure air, gave them an advantage in developing the beauty, strength, and health of their children, which it would be difficult to secure with our climate and habits,

And the steady and equable climate of the old countries, which has led their inhabitants to out-door life, and thus to acquire vigorous constitutions, gives them also a great advantage over us.

But then our difficulties *can* be met and overcome.

Every man who is a householder should be sure that every member of his family breathes pure air, not only all day but all night, by this simple arrangement: In every room of his house let at least one window be let down at the top two inches, and one door have an opening of two inches over the top. Let this be done in such a way that no person *can* alter it. For if ventilators are fixed so that they can be closed, they will be, in the majority of cases, by the ignorant, or timid, or falsely economical.

A house thus arranged will require more fuel to warm it, but the additional expense of this will not be a tenth part of that which would result from the loss of labor and health consequent on the debility and disease always resulting, more or less, from the habitual inhalation of impure air.

In a house thus arranged, stoves—though less healthful than open fires—would still be far less injurious than they now are.

And here one common prejudice against "night-air," resulting solely from ignorance, must be met.

It has been shown that every pair of lungs vitiates a hogshead of air every hour, by withdrawing from it one half its oxygen, and replacing it with the same quantity of carbonic acid. Now, at night, the inmates of a house must either breathe pure air, that constantly flows in from without and thus drives out the impure air within, or they must keep on breathing over and over again the confined air of the house, that every hour grows more and more poisonous and debilitating.

The popular objections to night-air are, that it is cold, or damp, or loaded with unhealthful miasmata. But if a person has bed-clothing enough to keep warm, the colder the air the better every way. And if the air is damp, so as to render the atmosphere of the room damp also, still no harm is done, *provided the body is kept warm.* Remember that the most delicate patients in health establishments sleep for hours with wet sheets packed around them, without the least evil or danger. A damp night-air never can harm the most delicate person if every part of the body is covered so as to be duly warm. As to the effect of damp air taken into the lungs, well educated people know that there is no time when there is more water held suspended in the atmosphere than in a hot day. When the air becomes cold this dampness becomes sensible to the eye and feeling, but there is really not so much water inhaled into the lungs in breathing a cold, damp air, as in breathing a warm and apparently dry atmosphere.

No reason, then, exists for excluding the night-air from the lungs when cold and damp; but more clothing is required, and more care to avoid a draft on any exposed part of the body. Of course, where lungs are diseased, any extremes in temperature must be avoided.

As to unhealthful miasmata in the night-air, nothing can be worse than the exhalations of decaying bodies, as sent forth from the lungs and skin of sleepers. It is precisely the same evil as is found in proximity to grave-yards and decaying carrion. The effluvium from the lungs and skin is precisely the same as that from carrion, only more diluted by the atmosphere. Those who have entered the pent-up sleeping rooms of persons who do not wash their skins or breathe a pure air, very well understand the close resemblance.

In the summer season, while vegetation is in life, it is true that the leaves of all trees and plants are *respiring;* giving out oxygen and taking in carbonic acid by day, and then at night throwing out carbonic acid and taking in oxygen. But this respiration of vegetable nature outside of our dwellings, and all the effluvia of decaying vegetation at any period of the year, are never so effective in destroying the healthfulness of the air around our dwellings, as the lungs of the inhabitants within them.

Let it also be considered that the air we do breathe—unless the house is air-tight, which no house can be—must be night-air, more or less mixed with the portion which has been breathed over and over again through the day and evening. So that every body *does* breathe night-air, or what is worse,

These things are presented in order to remove that baleful prejudice and fear that so many ignorant persons indulge toward their best friends, *air and water*.

To return : let every person who has charge of a family make some *sure* arrangement thus to secure to every person in their house an abundance of pure air for their lungs and skin both by day and night, and the grand cause that, above all others, is gradually deteriorating the vigor, health, and beauty of the American people will disappear.

Add to this, appropriate care that all the school-rooms in the land have the same arrangement made to provide pure air for the pupils. Keep the tops of the windows down both in winter and summer, and pay for the increase of fuel instead of the doctor and grave-digger.   In every community where there are colleges and seminaries, as well as the public schools, there ought to be inspectors appointed, the same as other civil officers, to go around and see whether any parent or teacher is poisoning the rising generation with impure air.   Oh, how many families, and schools, and boarding establishments have come within my circuit in which this evil, even to this hour, is perpetuated !

No parents, no guardians of the young should ever retire to rest till fully assured that every one under their care is furnished with the full supply of pure air for the night. And all employers, in all kinds of business, should be taught that they are committing a great sin against the life and welfare of those they employ, if they force them to labor in impure air.   Every minister of the gospel should, in the first place take care that his own spiritual concerns, and those of his hearers are not checked and interrupted by brains stupefied by bad air ; and next, he should teach his people their obligations in this matter, both to themselves and to all under their care.   The physician, too, is especially bound to use all his influence in a community in the same direction.

EXERCISE AND AMUSEMENT.

Next to pure air, *healthful exercise and amusements* are the most important remedies for the evils set forth.

The modes for securing these are not so easily indicated.   A great part of the American people exercise certain portions of their muscular system too much, while their intellect has little activity, and their spirits are rarely cheered and animated by amusements. Another portion keep their brain in constant labor, without the balancing influence of muscular activity, or the relief of recreation. And still another portion give up their whole being to pleasure-seeking and amusement, without any useful activity either of body or mind.

There are various measures which might be adopted, that each in its place would tend to a better adjustment of this difficult matter. To illustrate what *might* be done, let it be imagined that, for the sake of an experiment, funds were provided, and the inhabitants of a community should all agree to give the method here suggested a fair trial.

In the first place, a course of lectures should be given, for the purpose of making the people fully understand the evils to be remedied, and the benefits to be secured.

Next, a central site should be provided, on which should be erected a large and beautiful building—a *Temple of Health.* Around it should be every variety of pleasant walks, and shades, and flowers, to attract and please in the summer months, and other arrangements provided for out-door sports and exercises in winter. Within the building should be arranged a great variety of apparatus and accommodations for in-door amusements that *exercise the muscles,* and those which in most cases could be performed *in measures and to the sound of music.* These exercises should be under the direction of scientific and medical men, and no one should be admitted to these premises except on condition that they would strictly obey the direction of these managers.

All persons attending should then be examined in regard to their daily avocations, their diet, the ventilation of their sleeping and business rooms, the defects of their physical system, and any disease they may suffer, and advice appropriate be given. Then a course of exercise, fitted to each case, should be marked out, and superintendents appointed to see that all these directions are obeyed. The aim should be, not only to secure exercise, but that kind which is appropriate to each case, and also that which would prove *exhilarating* and *amusing.* For exercise that is sought as a pleasure is more than doubled in value.

In short, every arrangement should be made in strict conformity to the laws of health, and all excess should be excluded. Here, too, parents should be instructed in family plays and games, and thus induced to join with their children in home amusements. For nothing so binds the young to those who control them, as aid and sympathy in amusing sports.

It is believed that if any community would once fairly test such a plan as this for six months, nine-tenths of the diseases, infirmities, low spirits, and ill-temper of that place would vanish away, while every social, domestic, and religious virtue would take a new start.

The preceding method is suggested mainly with reference to adults. In regard to the rising generation, the grand remedy must be in connection with schools and other institutions for education.

As these are now conducted, all the money, time, and efforts are spent in training and exercising the intellect. In our higher institutions, one department is *endowed* that a teacher may give all his time and efforts to cultivating the mathematical faculties. Another endowment supports a teacher to train the linguistic powers. Another endowment secures a teacher for chemistry—another provides for some other of the natural sciences. Thus, there is a constantly accumulating outlay for divisions and subdivisions of labor, and all for the intellectual department of education. Stringent rules also are made, and laws enforced to secure obedience to arrangements that often involve most flagrant violations of the laws of health.

But where in the wide circuit of our nation is an institution where even *one* teacher is sustained, whose official duty it is to secure the health and perfect development of that wonderful and curious organism on which the mind is so dependent? Why should not the students in our colleges and other institutions of learning be required to breathe pure air; to exercise their muscles appropriately and sufficiently; to retire as well as to rise at proper hours; to take care of the skin, and to avoid the use of stimulating herbs and drinks? And why should not endowments be provided to sustain a well qualified and able man, whose official duty it shall be to give instructions, and exercise the supervision that would secure so important a result?

In regard to all our common and other schools for young children, to the proper ventilation of their school-rooms should be added a complete and scientific training of their bodies to perfect health and the full development of every part. This is entirely practicable, and would be immediately adopted by every teacher did the public demand it. One half hour of every school session ought to be spent by every teacher and pupil in a regular course of calisthenic and gymnastic exercises, that should be as imperative as any other school duty.

A universal course of training of this kind, scientifically arranged and applied, in connection with obedience to other laws of health, might, in one generation, transform the inhabitants of this land from the low development now so extensive to the beautiful model of the highest form of humanity.

Children, too, can be made to understand all that is contained in this book as to the construction of their own bodies and the laws of health. And such knowledge is as important for them, in order to secure their obedience to these laws, as it is for grown persons. Nothing can be made more interesting to children than information in regard to the curious construction of their own bodies; while this alone will secure an intelligent and cheerful submission to rules that regulate their appetites and propensities.

FOOD AND DRINK.

Next in importance to air and exercise comes the selection of diet and drink. And in this matter the practical adoption of one common-sense maxim would do almost all that needs to be done. The maxim is this: *In cases where one of two courses involves danger and risk and another is perfectly safe, always choose the path of safety.*

We have seen that the great mass of this nation is fast hastening to disease and deterioration, and that individual misery and domestic unhappiness are widely increasing as the result. We have seen that owing to needless varieties, to stimulating food and drinks, and to the use of condiments, *excess* in loading the digestive organs is one great cause of this extensive suffering.

Now there is a rich variety and abundance of simple, healthful food and drinks that are fitted for the perfect development and nutrition of the body, and involve little liability to perversion and excess.   And when all stimulating food, drinks, and condiments are relinquished and a simple diet maintained, a *healthful appetite* returns, which is a safe guide to the proper amount to be taken, provided always that enough pure air and exercise are secured.

Moreover, I have found by my own experience, and have learned from others, that after living for several months on simple food, there is an increased susceptibility of taste and a keener relish for the delicate flavors that simple food offers.   Does any one remember the delicious relish of childhood for a bit of good bread?   This same relish will again return when solicited aright.   Let a person for several weeks try the experiment of drinking only water, eating nothing but bread and butter, potatoes, baked fruit, and milk, and at the same time exercise abundantly in the fresh air, and if their experience corresponds with that of most I have known who have tried the experiment, they will say, "Never did food of the richest variety and composition furnish such an exquisite relish!"

The more a person will limit a meal to *a few articles*, and these of the *simplest kind*, the more will they regain the appetite and relish of early life.

Now the course here suggested is perfectly safe, is equally productive of enjoyment, and is in obedience to the laws of health, which are the laws of God.   The common course pursued in this land of abundance and gormandizing is certainly one of risk and danger to the delicate and deteriorated constitutions of the adult and rising generations.   Is not here the place to practice the Christian "daily" duty of "self-denial?"   And if the strong and healthy feel no need of it for themselves, is there not a duty set forth for them in this inspired command, "We that are strong ought to bear the infirmities of the weak, and not to please ourselves?"

In reference to stimulating drinks, how often have I seen

the need of this divine injunction. The parents of a family drink strong tea and coffee. They teach their children perhaps, that it is a dangerous and unhealthy practice, and train them to entire abstinence. But after a few years these children draw to manhood and womanhood, and begin to claim the privileges of acting by their own judgments. Then, after a period of deprecation and remonstrance, the luxury is conceded. Some one of the flock is weak, the strong can bear it but the weak one falters. No eye but that of the Heavenly Parent marks how this one single cause is daily draining the already stinted nervous fountain. And when the flower is cut down, the weeping parents mourn over the sacrifice offered by themselves to their own self-indulgence—to their neglect of that beneficent law, "We that are strong ought to bear the infirmities of the weak, and not to please ourselves."

Oh, tender parents, who provide these dangerous beverages, look around your beloved circle and see which one you can select as the hapless victim!

And so in reference to that disgusting and baleful use of tobacco, which all over the nation is draining the nervous fountain of thousands of pale and delicate young men. The clergyman, the church elder, the father of the family, indulge in a useless and dangerous practice, merely to gratify a morbid appetite. While they teach others to " deny fleshly lusts," and upbraid the young if they fall, in their own cherished fleshly appetite they see no sin, because they say it does not hurt *themselves*.

But every young victim to this appetite who has been led on by their example, or has not been withheld when their arguments and example might have saved them, is set down to their account by Him who seeth not as man seeth. He whose example of self-denying benevolence they profess to follow, whose last teachings on earth were, " If ye love me feed my sheep; feed my lambs"—He has left to them, above all others, the sacred monition, "We that are strong ought to bear the infirmities of the weak, and not to please ourselves."

In regard to the use of tobacco, it seems to me the American people, for want of a little consideration, are invading their high character for respectful kindness and deference to woman. In this matter, there are few that have so much occasion as myself to render a grateful acknowledgment of this most chivalrous virtue in my countrymen; for during the last period of my life I have crossed from West to East, or from East to West, not less than thirty times, and have traveled in all the Free States and five of the Southern; and in all this varied experience, when, in a large portion of the cases also, I was without a protector, I have never *once* known of a coarse or disrespectful word or act toward myself, or witnessed one toward any other woman. At the same time, all that father or brother could render has been accorded by strangers.

But in my recent travels, especially at the West, I have constantly been made to feel what a *selfish* as well as disgusting and ungallant habit is induced by the use of tobacco! The majority of ladies are offended by the effluvium of that weed, and disgusted by its marks on the mouth and face, while the puddles of tobacco juice that infest our public conveyances, the breath of smokers, and the wads and squirting of chewers, not only defile the dress but keep a sensitive stomach in constant excitement and agitation. There have been times in my experience when it seemed to me I must give up a journey from this cause alone. Certainly, if those who practice this vice will insist on perfuming public conveyances with dead tobacco smoke from their dress and lungs, and rendering all their premises filthy and disgusting with their expectorations, the managers of these conveyances should provide rooms and cars for ladies and all other persons who are annoyed by this vice, from which all who either smoke or chew shall be excluded.

LETTER TWENTY-FOURTH.

NEXT to air, exercise, and diet, the care of that complicated and sensitive organ *the skin* is to be regarded.

Under this head will be placed also what is to be said on the subject of *dress* and *deformities*.

In regard to the care of the skin, it has been shown that the full circulation of blood in its capillaries, and the free discharge of its secretions, are the objects to be aimed at in promoting perfect health. For this purpose air, light, water, friction, and cold are the chief agencies, and are also healthful tonics to the nervous system generally, from its intimate connection with the skin.

All these agencies are secured by a daily morning ablution of the whole person. In order to this, no extensive bathing apparatus is required. A screen, made like a small clothes-frame, to set around a wash-stand, a bowl of cold water, and two towels, are all that are needed.

The quickest way to bathe is, with one towel, dipped in water, to wet first the upper and then the lower portions of the body, and then to rub them till dry and red with the other towel, which should be a rough and coarse one.

This followed by drinking two tumblers of cold water and a walk in the cool morning air, or, when the weather forbids, a series of *calisthenic* exercises before an open window, will give a healthful glow and appetite.

As to dress, it should always be sufficient in thickness and warmth to prevent any sense of uncomfortable chilliness. This being secured, the less clothing the better for the skin and the whole body.

Heat is always debilitating to the skin, while cold and

pure air are tonics. But all changes in this particular must be gradual, and great care must be taken not to exceed the nervous supply of the system, by abstracting animal heat too often and too long.

A great many persons lose all the benefits of water-treatment, and others bring on disease, by not understanding the importance of this caution.

In regard to the fashion of dress, it always should be so loose as to allow the *fullest* inspiration of the lungs without any consequent pressure. Every mantua-maker should be required to take her measures when the lungs are entirely filled.

As for striving to make women dress " out of the fashion," in order to be healthy, the effort would be folly and a failure. The wiser way is to circumvent Madam Fashion by contrivances that shall in the main pay her all demanded deference, and yet conform to the rules of health and decency.

The present style, which demands that the middle portion of the female form be drawn in like the body of a wasp, while the lower portion must flare out like an umbrella, can be secured without the disgusting and murderous methods the results of which will now be again presented.

On the next page are two figures, one of which represents the waist of the most perfect model of a beautiful female form. The other represents the fashionable waist of modern days, which can be achieved only by deforming the bones, and displacing the most delicate and important internal organs.

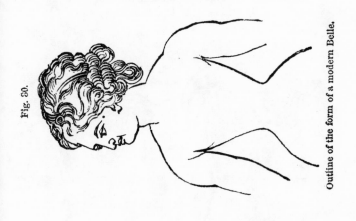

Fig. 30.

Outline of the form of a modern Belle.

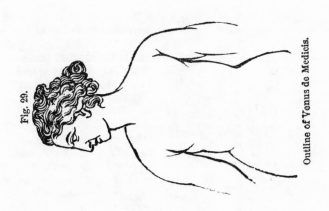

Fig. 29.

Outline of Venus de Medicis.

M

Here is a drawing of the skeletons of these female figures—the one as Nature designed it, and the other as Art deforms it.

Fig. 81.

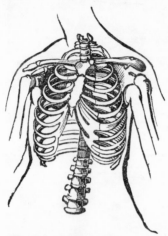

Fig. 82.

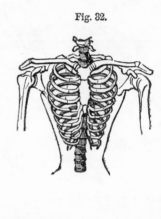

The skeleton as Nature formed it.   The skeleton as deformed by Art.

The poor young girl whom the mother is dressing for a

Fig. 33.

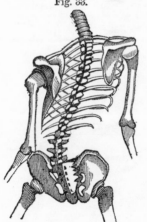

sacrifice to this horrid fashion, remorselessly girds the waist just where the bones have least internal support and yield the easiest. The small floating ribs are pressed unequally and laterally against the spine, because the intestines can not yield the equal support required. The result is a distortion of this kind. Fig. 33.

Any mother can discover when this deformity is secured by examining these drawings—Fig. 34 showing the external appearance of the back as Nature designed it should be, and

Fig. 35 the deformity caused by tight dress.   These views are presented, because in many cases this evil, if discovered soon enough, can be remedied by methods to be hereafter indicated.

Fig. 34.

Fig. 35.

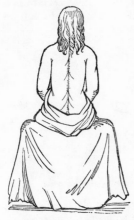
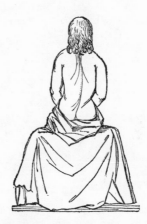

The same deformity of the spine is sometimes caused or increased by wrong positions in sleeping.   If the body is placed in a perfectly horizontal position—as may be seen in the drawing at Fig. 36—all pressure is taken from the car-

Fig. 36.

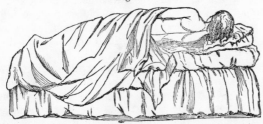

tilage discs of the spine, and thus, for seven or eight hours out of the twenty-four, they are enabled gradually to return to their natural form.   It is found by measurement that, in this way, the spine is every night *lengthened*—these discs re-

·covering by their elasticity a slight increase of thickness. Thus, every person is a little taller in the morning than at night.

But when a person sleeps with a high pillow, so that the spine is bent through the night, this relieving process is not allowed to certain portions of the spinal discs. (Here is a drawing, Fig. 37, to illustrate.) The result is, in certain

Fig. 37.

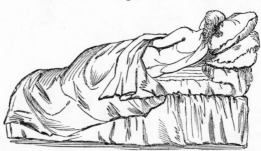

cases where delicacy of constitution particularly affects the bony portion of the body, that the spine becomes more or less distorted. This shows why it is that children should not be allowed high pillows. The pillow should be just high enough to keep the head in the natural position; and the child should be taught to sleep on both sides, if there is any danger of a departure from this ordinary practice.

Another, and still more frequent mode of distorting the spine is by the positions that children assume at school, or in study and writing at home. The drawing (Fig. 38 and Fig. 39) on the opposite page represents the right and the wrong methods of sitting when drawing and writing. When children sit on high benches so that their feet can not rest on the floor, when they are obliged to sit long with the back unsupported, and when they bend over to study and read, the muscles that hold the body in its proper position become exhausted, the discs of the spine gradually harden, and various deformities—such as projecting necks, round shoulders, and crooked backs—are the result. In childhood, and often among adults, most of these deform-

Fig. 38.   Fig. 39.

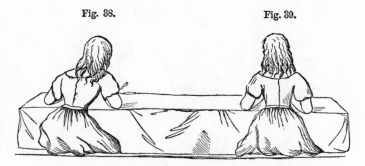

ities can be remedied by methods to be hereafter indicated.

But, as has been before shown, the most terrible evil that mischievous fashions in dress have induced is the internal displacements and change of form exhibited in the article furnished by Mrs. Gleason. These are caused by the combined influence of *tight* dress, pressing the central organs downward on the lower ones, and the debility and pressure induced by the *heat* and *weight* of clothing around the hips. Let the reader again examine, in the beginning of that article, the beautiful curves of the chest and spine of the perfect form, as viewed sidewise, and then compare it with the distorted one.

Then notice the outline of a healthy, finely-formed child, and see how it entirely corresponds, in a side view, with this drawing of a perfect form. Then notice most of the female forms in a drawing-room, and see how many there are that sink *inward* in front, instead of showing the beautiful *outward* curve. The effort to gain the "slender waist," which novelists and dress-makers set forth to admiration, as the Chinese do the stump foot, often produces this outward distortion, with little consciousness of the still more shocking internal results.

Now, it is to circumvent Madam Fashion in this, the climax of her murderous follies, that a fashion of under-garments is suggested, which is illustrated in Fig. 40 and Fig. 41, on page 182.

Fig. 40.   Fig. 41.

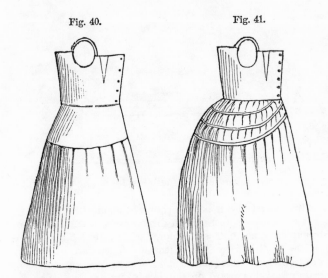

Fig. 40 shows the outline of a warm, close *under*-petti-coat, in which there is no accumulation of plaits or gathers around the waist, and the design of which is to keep the body *equally* warm in all parts. The fullness in this case is made at the lower line, as shown by the drawing. At the same time, by waist and shoulder-straps, the weight is borne by the shoulders, and the upper part of the body is dressed as warm as the lower.

But our second drawing (Fig. 41) is our main achieve-ment in circumventing the evils of the present fashion. By this method a woman can spread out her robes below, to any extent she may deem necessary in order to secure her the very pinnacle of fashionable expansion. In this drawing, a waist is made which rests by straps on the shoulders, and to which the skirt below can be buttoned. The skirt is made of two parts. The upper is a long, double strip, with *slides* made in it for inserting whalebones, as is done in drawn bonnets. Then this strip is drawn up on these whalebones till it assumes the form of that part of a fash-ionable lady where from six to twelve skirts ordinarily are sustained, weighing from four to six or eight pounds. Then the lower portion of the petticoat is to be gathered or plaited on to this, and the whole fastened to the waist by buttons.

By this method a skirt is made that can expand to any dimensions, and yet be light and cool for summer. Then when cold weather comes, the added clothing can nestle under its broad expanse. By this method, too, a lady can appear in the height of the mode, and yet, so far as this matter is concerned, violate none of the laws of health.

CUSTOMS OF SOCIAL LIFE.

The American people claim to be in advance of all other nations in civil and religious liberty. They are complimented as the people who are to take the lead in guiding all others to the most perfect state of social, civil, and moral development.

If this honorable career is before them, it surely is inconsistent with their high vocation to become slaves to injurious customs that are manufactured for them abroad. Why should not the American people originate customs in social life as much in advance of old nations as are their civil concerns?

We have seen that *light* is more favorable to health and perfect development than darkness. We have seen that even the trees and shrubs that exhale their life-inspiring oxygen by day and their carbon through the night, are teaching mankind that the time for the quick circulation of muscular labor and of brain excitement is *the day*, while the slow breath of slumber is reserved for the less healthful atmosphere of night.

Now those countries whose customs are founded on the assumption that one class of people are to do the work and another class are to appropriate the best fruits of this labor, have instituted social customs on the plan of making every possible barrier of separation between these two classes. And so the aristocracy sit up all night and sleep by day, while those who carry on the business of the world are abroad in the light and slumber in the hours appointed by God for sleep.

But it is the pride of our nation that all men are equal in rights and privileges, and that no aristocracy can flourish here. Why, then, should we not banish those customs of social life that are low imitations of what is false and wrong? Why should not the American people set an example to the Old World of customs conformed at once to the laws of health, the laws of God, and the spirit of their own boasted institutions?

In the palmy days of our early Republic, all classes rose with the sun, and all the hours of labor, even for the highest, were by daylight. And their social gatherings were ordinarily ended when the "nine o'clock bell" gave warning that all well-ordered families should retire to rest.

In another matter we have an opportunity to excel even the fathers of our Republic. The farther man advances from childhood and in social life from the savage state, the more do refined and intellectual pleasures take the place of merely animal. In the lower states of society the chief attractions to social gatherings were *eating and drinking*. But just in proportion as man becomes elevated, this lowest species of enjoyment gives place to higher and more refined pleasure.

May we not hope that our country is so far advanced as to be able to institute new customs in these respects? Can not the principle of "association," which accomplishes so many other social improvements, be brought to bear upon this matter?

It certainly is true that the great body of cultivated and sensible people in this country heartily despise and condemn the vulgar gatherings where a good part of the night is spent in unhealthful air, unhealthful dresses, stupid recognitions, and unseasonable eating and drinking. Why should this sensible portion be controlled by the uncultivated and frivolous? Why should not the really "best circles" associate on the principles of common sense, democracy, and Christianity, and agree to have their social gatherings such as are worthy of our country and our country's "best society," and such as we may set forth as examples of a higher civilization to all other nations?

LETTER TWENTY-FIFTH.

IN pointing out what is to be done, there are certain classes who have a prominent interest and responsibility in regard to this effort. Among the foremost are the really well-educated members of the medical profession of all schools.

It is *knowledge among the people* in regard to the wonderful and complicated mechanism of their own bodies, that alone can secure to properly qualified physicians that respect and confidence which is now so extensively shared by ignorant presumers. And thus it is, that any effort to enlighten the people is one in which such physicians have alike a personal, a professional, and a philanthropic interest.

The ministers of religion also have a deep concern in this undertaking. There is such an intimate connection between body and spirit that one can not deteriorate and fail without involving the other. Diseased and debilitated nerves are probably the cause of as much sin as they are of suffering. Thousands of cases of spiritual stupidity or darkness would be effectually remedied by restoring health and healthful avocations.

If the ministers of religion would learn themselves what the laws of health are, and obey them—if they would set them forth as the *laws of God*—if they would teach their people that they commit sin when they violate these laws, as really as when they swear, or steal, or break the Sabbath —if the solemn sanctions of the eternal world were brought to bear on the conscience in reference to these obligations as they are in regard to what are distinctly taught as religious duties, there would be an immense and most healthful influence emanating from the pulpit which now is almost entirely wanting.

While the clergy and medical profession can exert an influence chiefly on adults, it is the teachers of schools, colleges, and professional institutions that hold an ·equal responsibility in regard to the coming generation. Such have daily opportunities of setting a good example themselves, while at the same time they can explain and enforce the obligations of the laws of health with great efficiency.

But it is woman, to whom, as wife, mother, educator, nurse, and house-keeper, the training of the human body in infancy and the ministries of the sick-room are specially committed, who has the most direct and immediate interest and responsibility in this effort.

Woman is the Heaven-appointed guardian of health in the family, as the physician is in the community; and though her duties are not as extensive or as complicated, they are more minute and constant, and equally important. Every woman, then, should regard this department of her duties as a part of her *profession*, for which she should be properly trained, and to which she should direct her earnest interest and attention.

From my own sex, then, I would especially seek attention to certain *details* where their influence may be brought to bear most efficiently.

I would ask every woman whose eye meets this page if she will consider her power of influence, and her consequent obligations under the several heads which these queries may suggest.

In the first place, then, will you, my friend, consider what you can do to save all around you from the destructive influence of a poisoned atmosphere? Will you examine all the sleeping rooms of the house you are in, and see if children and servants, as well as the parents, have a full supply of pure air, not only all day, but *all night?* And if they do not, will you direct attention to what this work offers on the subject, and use all your influence to have the evil remedied?

And if you have access to those who have clerks, apprentices, or laborers under their charge, will you direct their attention to this matter, which is so seldom considered. And when you visit the poor, will you seek to instruct them on this subject, and point out any injurious practices you may observe in this respect?

Will you observe whether your churches and lecture-rooms are properly ventilated, and if not, use your influence to remedy the neglect? And will you protest in all suitable ways against the unhealthful mode of construction in traveling accommodations?

In regard to *exercise*, which comes next in importance to pure air, will you lend all your influence to elevate the dignity and promote the agreeableness and good taste of *domestic labor*. God made woman to do the work of the family state, and all her *physique* is exactly adapted to her duties. And all the arrangements of the family should be such as to make household employment honorable, tasteful, and agreeable. A woman's kitchen and nursery ought to be the two pleasantest rooms in the house, and more pains should be taken to make them attractive than is now given to ornament the parlor. A house perfectly ventilated, with all its inhabitants engaged in the exercises of domestic labor, is the *beau-ideal* of the family state.

But when riches come, a style of living *will* come that demands servants; and when there are servants enough to do all the labor, the women and children *will not work*. Then the next best thing is a system of *calisthenics*, that shall be made a regular part of school training for children, while adults should have gymnastic assembly-rooms for similar purposes. But every man, woman, and child in the nation, ought to spend one or two hours every day in *vigorous* exercise of *all* the muscles. Will you lend your influence to promote this?

In regard to *dress*, will you lend all your influence to end the murderous practices that are ruining and distorting the female form all over the nation? Will you furnish mantua-makers with this volume to read, and urge on them their responsibilities in this direction? Will those of you who have access to the originators and publishers of our *fashion plates*, use your influence to modify the baneful consequences that flow from this source? Will you take care that every young girl under your control dresses loosely, has all the weight of her clothing rest on her shoulders, and does not accumulate an excess of clothing on any portion of the person?

Will you promote a simple and healthful diet, not banishing *variety*, but having it *successive* instead of heaping it all together at one meal. Will you use your influence to banish all stimulating condiments and stimulating drinks? Especially, will you discountenance the use of tobacco, which is now ruining the health and tempting to inebriety thousands of the flower of our youth?

Will you lend your influence to promote a reform in social gatherings? This can be done most effectually by those who take the lead in fashion. But in every place a few families might change the customs by a little consultation and agreement.

If some of the more influential families in a community will decide that their social gatherings shall be at proper hours, and that the dress, entertainment, and amusements shall all conform to the laws of health, the evils that arise from this source would be ended in that sphere, and gradually others would adopt the same customs.

ASSOCIATION OF AMERICAN WOMEN.

This is the age in which almost every important or benevolent undertaking is carried forward by the power of *association*. Among the multitudes of enterprises that thus demand public attention, has appeared an organization to secure "the rights" and redress "the wrongs" of woman.

While conceding to those who conduct this effort the best of motives, and great talent and skill in promoting their aims, and while it is impossible not to sympathize with them in some of the particulars for which they labor, yet, as a whole, their undertaking seems based on a false view of the true duties and interests of woman in the social state.

It is evident that Providence designed that the chief responsibility of *sustaining the family state*, in all its sacred and varied relations and duties, should rest mainly on the female sex. In the perfected state of human society, toward which we hope our nation is to be the leader, as a general rule, every man will be able to support a family and will seek a wife. In such a condition of society, the nursing and educating of children, the care of the sick, and the various departments of domestic economy, which all will allow are better filled by women than by men, will demand all the women there are. In such a state, all can see that it would be folly to entice woman into the business and professions of man.

But in seeking to remedy the misadjustments and abuses of society which bear severely on woman, is it not equally unwise to adopt a course—unless, perhaps, as a temporary expedient to relieve immediate suffering—which is directly antagonistic to the true pattern that eventually we hope to see accomplished? Instead of combining to entice woman into new professions, and those as yet exclusively held by man, it is deemed wiser to aim rather to retain her in her own most appropriate sphere, by rendering it so attractive and honorable, that she can not improve her condition by forsaking it.

It was in such a view of the case that some years ago an organization of ladies was commenced in New York city, which has quietly been seeking to promote the interests of woman by measures and aims that it was supposed would meet the approbation of American women of all sects and parties.

The *name* of this organization is the *American Woman's Educational Association.* Its *object,* as stated in its Constitution, is "to aid in securing to American women a liberal education, honorable position, and remunerative employment *in their appropriate profession;* the distinctive profession of woman being considered as embracing the training of the human mind, the care of the human body in infancy and sickness, and the conservation of the family state."

"The *leading measure* to be pursued by the Association is the establishment of permanent *endowed* institutions for women;" the "endowments" being employed "to furnish the salaries of three superior teachers in each institution, who shall take charge of the three departments set forth as constituting *the profession of woman.*"

The *mode* in which this effort has been carried out, has been to seek the co-operation of a large town or city in founding such an institution, by the offer, on the part of the Association, of a library and apparatus, and a permanent endowment of *twenty thousand dollars* for the above purpose, on condition that the citizens erect a suitable building, and insure an income from tuition fees that will support four teachers for the literary departments.

This offer was made to the citizens of Milwaukee, Wisconsin, and of Dubuque, Iowa. The result has been the erection, in each of these cities, of a large and beautiful edifice for such an institution. In Milwaukee about two hundred pupils, and in Dubuque nearly one hundred, are in a course of study in the institutions thus established.

It is now the object of the Association to organize the three departments in these institutions, which are to be sustained by *endowment*, and which aim to qualify woman for her *distinctive duties*. These are, first, the Normal Department, where the pupils are to be trained to act as educators; next, the Health Department, where they are to be trained to be perfectly healthy themselves, and to understand all that appertains to the care of infancy and of family health; and, lastly, the Domestic Department, where they are to be trained to understand and perform all the processes of domestic economy.

Those who superintend this enterprise believe that far more can be accomplished in these departments of female education than has ever yet been attempted. And though there may be difficulties and prejudices to overcome, this is the common lot of all great and good undertakings. They have a plan, which they believe can be carried out, and they hope not only to secure the results aimed at in the institutions under their immediate patronage, but so to establish the practicability and value of the method, that it will be eventually adopted by other female institutions throughout the land.

In this enterprise, the part which has absorbed my chief interest has been that which relates to *health*. And inasmuch as one of the heaviest drains on the life and health of American women is owing to their imperfect training for the complicated duties of domestic economy, this is regarded as scarcely separable from the other.

With reference to the organization of the Health Departments, a work has been prepared by me, entitled,

PHYSIOLOGY AND CALISTHENICS FOR COMMON SCHOOLS. This work will contain all that is embraced, on physiology and the laws of health, in the two first portions of these Letters, arranged in lessons to be recited at school. Connected with this will be a course of *Calisthenic Training* for the young of both sexes, arranged on scientific principles, for the perfect development of a healthful body, and illustrated by drawings. In preparing this work, the system of *Ling*, the Swedish philanthropist, and all accessible works relating to this subject, have been studied, while all that has been gained by the experience of Health Establishments has also been made available.

One portion of this work will embrace those exercises which have been found to be so successful in rectifying deformities and relieving disease, and which are specially serviceable in health establishments.

The way is now prepared to indicate one mode by which American women, by methods more or less formal, may *associate* to promote the best interest of their own sex, and thus of the whole commonwealth.

The copyright interest of these Letters, and of the work on Physiology and Calisthenics, and also of a small work on Geography for Schools, presented by my sister, Mrs. H. B. Stowe, for the same object, are transferred to the Trustees of the American Woman's Educational Association, to be held in trust for that Association.

By the terms of agreement with the publishers of these works (Harper and Brothers, New York, and Phillips and Sampson, Boston), *half the net profits* on all sales made by booksellers will be paid to the Trustees of this Association. In addition to this, the agents of the Association, and committees of ladies acting for the purpose, are to be furnished with these works by the publishers *at cost*. By this method *the whole* of the profits will accrue to the Association on all sales made through their agents and committees.

That is to say, when these books are bought at book-stores *half* the net profits goes to the Association ; but when bought of the agents *the whole* net profit belongs to the Association.

Inasmuch as several well-dressed women in various parts of the country have raised money on false pretenses as my agents, I would caution the public to discredit all such claims unless sustained by abundant credentials. No committee, agent, or bookseller will be authorized by me or by the Association for this object except with my signature. The amount received by the Association from this source will be published in their Annual Report.

To facilitate purchases from the agents and committees, this work is done up in a form to send *by mail*, and any person who will transmit to me any sum not less than a dollar shall receive the value in copies of this work at the retail price at which it could be bought at book-stores, and with no other expense. When an Association is formed to aid in circulating this work, and in advancing the whole enterprise, larger quantities can be sent to them by Express.

Orders may be sent, *addressed to me personally*, and my agents will attend to them punctually. In order to accommodate different sections, my addresses for this purpose are:

Dr. BAILEY, Editor of the *National Era*, Washington.

Rev. Dr. T. BRAINERD, Philadelphia.

WILLIAM A. BEECHER, New York.

Rev. Dr. EDWARD BEECHER, Boston.

JOHN P. FOOTE, Esq., Cincinnati.

O. H. WALDO, Esq., Milwaukee, Wisconsin.

Those wishing to aid the object by this method, should address me at the place among these which is nearest their residence.

It is the aim of the ladies who already are associated in this enterprise, so far as is possible, to secure t*he reading of these Letters* by every man and woman in this nation who can understand them, and to enlist in the effort the co-operation, not only of their own sex, but of their clergymen, physicians, and editorial friends. As one result of this measure, they hope to secure the introduction of the work on *Physiology and Calisthenics* into schools of all descriptions all over the land, and thus to promote a great improvement in the physical training of the next generation. This last work will not be ready for sale till October, 1855.

The following are the Board of Managers and the Trustees of the American Woman's Educational Association.

BOARD OF MANAGERS

OF THE AMERICAN WOMAN'S EDUCATIONAL ASSOCIATION.

N

NOTES.

Note I.

The following is furnished by Mrs. R. B. Gleason, of the Elmira Water Cure, N. Y. This lady is a regularly educated physician, and has practiced, in connection with her husband, for ten years, confining her attention chiefly to patients of her own sex. She first studied with her husband, who is a graduate of the medical school at Castleton, Vermont. Afterward she took two courses of medical lectures at two of the small number of medical schools that allow these advantages to women, and received her diploma. In this lady are united more than ordinary talents, sound common-sense, benevolence, and refinement.

ELMIRA WATER CURE, N. Y., *April* 15, 1855.

DEAR MADAM—The following views and facts, drawn up at your request, I forward for you to use in any way that may promote the benevolent objects at which you are aiming. I will arrange them, as you desire, under the following heads: 1. Internal displacements and disorders connected with them. 2. Necessity for local mechanical treatment. 3. Symptoms of pelvic displacement and diseases and their treatment. 4. Effects of imagination in reference to these diseases. 5. Effects of these complaints on character and domestic happiness. 5. Peculiar instructions needed by young children. 7. Instructions at a more mature age. 8. Deterioration of women.

1. *Internal Displacements.*

To understand this portion it will be needful to examine the two drawings on next page, that represented at Fig. 42, *a side view* of a perfectly shaped body, and of the *packing* of the internal organs, and at Fig. 43, a distorted form, in which these organs have *sunk downward;* *h* is the heart, *d* the diaphragm, *S* the stomach. In the perfect form it is seen that the diaphragm curves, and the heart rests on it, while the stomach is supported by the intestines below it. Notice also the beautiful curve of the chest and spine. In the distorted form it is seen that the diaphragm has sunk to a nearly straight line, so that the heart is unsupported, while the stomach has lost its support by the falling of the abdominal viscera. Compare the two figures with both the perpendicular and the horizontal lines and notice the difference. This distortion is one of the results of *debility* and *tight-dresses*. The evils that result will now be indicated.

Fig. 42.   Fig. 43.

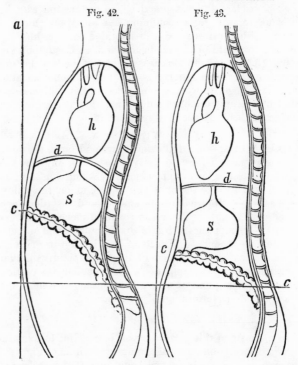

The internal organs, when closely folded and packed, must be strongly sustained both in front and below to keep

them in the natural form. This sustaining power is exerted
by what are called the *abdominal muscles*, which run upward, downward, and crosswise in front, their attachments
being to the breast-bone, hips, pelvic bones, and spine.
There are also muscles at the extreme base, within the pelvic cavity, that have a similar function.

The combined influences of bad air, bad food, excess in
eating, want of exercise, and excessive stimulus of the
brain and nerves, produce a general delicacy and debility
of the whole organism, in which the abdominal muscles
especially suffer.   They lose their vigor and elasticity, become flabby and easily stretched, without power to recover
their natural functions.   In this state of debility the present
style of dress has done every thing that can be done to de-
prive them of what little functional power would otherwise
have remained.   The result has been thousands and thousands of such distorted specimens of humanity as are exhibited in Fig. 43, on opposite page.   A really perfectly
formed woman, on the true model of beauty and proportion, designed by the Creator, and perpetuated in marble
statues by artists, is but rarely seen among our countrywo-
men.   Every woman who has a waist to correspond with
the fashion plates, usually has her interior organs in such
a shocking and disgusting situation as is here portrayed,
or is fast approximating toward it.

Disorders connected with these internal Displacements.

When, as has been shown, the abdominal muscles have
lost their power, the whole system of organs mainly resting
on them for support can not continue in their naturally
snug, compact, and rounded form, but become separated,
elongated, and unsupported.   The stomach begins to draw
from above instead of resting on the viscera beneath.   This
in some cases causes dull and wandering pains, a sense of
pulling at the centre of the chest, and a drawing downward
at the pit of the stomach.   Then as the support beneath is
really *gone*, there is what is often called "a feeling of *gone-
ness*," which is sometimes relieved by food which, so long as
it remains in a solid form, helps to hold up the falling su-
perstructure.   This displacement of the stomach, liver, and

spleen, interrupt their healthful functions, and dyspepsia and biliary difficulties not unfrequently are the result.

As the stomach and its appendages fall downward, the diaphragm with the heart and lungs, must descend also. In this state of things, the inflation of the lungs is less and less aided by the abdominal muscles, and is confined chiefly to the upper portion. Breathing sometimes thus becomes quicker and shorter on account of the elongated or debilitated condition of the assisting organs. Consumption not unfrequently results from this cause.

The heart also feels the evil. "Palpitations," "flutterings," "sinking feelings," all show that, in the language of Scripture, "the heart trembleth, and is moved out of its place."

But the lower intestines are the greatest sufferers from this dreadful abuse of nature. Having the weight of all the unsupported organs above pressing them into unnatural and distorted positions, the passage of the food is interrupted, and inflammations, indurations, and constipation, are the frequent result, and one in which both sexes are equal sufferers. Dreadful ulcers and cancers may be traced in some instances to this cause.

But this distortion brings on woman peculiar distresses. The pressure of the whole superincumbent mass on the pelvic organs induces sufferings proportioned in acuteness to the extreme delicacy and sensitiveness of the parts thus crushed. And the intimate connection of these organs with the brain and whole nervous system renders injuries thus inflicted the causes of the most extreme anguish, both of body and mind. This evil is becoming so common not only among married women, but among young girls, as is a just cause for universal alarm.

How very common these sufferings are, few but the medical profession can realize, because these are troubles that must be concealed. Many a woman is moving about in uncomplaining agony who, with any other complaint, involving equal suffering, would be on her bed surrounded by sympathizing friends.

2. *Local and Mechanical Treatment.*

It can not but be seen, even by the most unlearned in medical affairs, that such evils as are pictured in the drawing at the beginning of this article, can not be remedied by *taking medicines into the stomach.* If a bone is broken, no medicine can mend it, and *mechanical* means alone can effect a cure. So, after a certain amount of displacement of the internal organs, mechanical means must be employed to replace them.

This indicates the propriety of the method now extensively adopted in various health establishments.

In the first place, the patient is required to commence a strict obedience to all the laws of health—simple diet, pure air, hard beds, proper positions, by night and day, and a regular, systematic training to invigorate the whole of the muscular system by appropriate exercise. With this is combined the medical use of water as a tonic to the whole nervous and muscular system, and as promoting healthful constitutional changes.

In a majority of cases, where displacements are not extreme and chronic, this course will secure perfect health, and a restoration of misplaced organs by the recuperative power of nature thus aided and strengthened.

But, in bad cases, there must be added to all the above *surgical and mechanical treatment for replacing the disarranged organs.* And where inflammation and ulceration of the diseased organs have supervened, still more trying and painful operations must be resorted to.

But many physicians, who are not properly qualified to distinguish the various forms of uterine disease, are liable to attribute all pelvic pains to "prolapsus;" and, treating for this, not only fail to cure cases of inflammation, ulceration, and induration, but by their uncalled-for manipulations greatly aggravate these affections. *Many* cases of this description have come to my care, of which I will cite one as an example. A widowed mother of a family dependent on her care, had been confined to her bed for three years. Her physician pronounced hers a case of "prolapsus," and proceeded to manipulate to replace the organ, and also applied supporters. This gave great agony, and yet was persisted in for some time. She finally was brought to me on a bed. The speculum soon proved hers to be a case of ulceration and enlargement. Four months of surgical and water treatment restored her to perfect health.

On the subject of displacement of the pelvic organs all local treatment is useless, while the style of dress and unhealthful habits that caused the evil continue; for it must be remembered that the uterus is not held firmly by muscles, but only by loose ligaments of cellular tissue, and folds of the serous membrane. In a healthful state it is not firmly fixed, but has almost a floating position, being held in its proper place mainly by the pressure of the surrounding organs. Thus it is dependent on the healthy tone and condition of these organs. Hence daily efforts to replace it are of little avail till air, exercise, and healthful habits give tone and energy to the whole system. There are cases of extensive *anteversion* and *retroversion*, which demand both internal and external manipulation, and also artificial supporters; but, happily, such cases are *very rare*. The great majority of instances of prolapsus, unaccompanied by inflammatory or organic disease, can be cured by air, exercise, and water-treatment, without mechanical means.

At a recent period in my medical practice, I frequently received patients from establishments in which the physicians were celebrated for their success in pelvic diseases, and from them I learned the method pursued. This was duly tested, and in pursuance of this method *daily operations* for replacement, in cases of prolapsus uteri, were tried. But after full opportunities for experiment, my convictions have constantly increased that, as a general rule, this method is in most cases totally needless, and in many decidedly injurious. Other practitioners, who have made the same experiment, have arrived at the same conclusion. Some statistics of my experience the past year will illustrate this.

From January 1, 1854, to January 1, 1855, there have been under my care for complaints of this description, *one hundred and thirty cases*. Of these *seventy-five* received no *local* treatment of any kind, though at least one-third of them suffered from weakness in the back and pelvic pains. These were all entirely cured by air, exercise, and water-treatment.

Fifty-seven received speculum treatment for either inflammation, or ulceration, or induration of the uterus.   Of these, *thirty-seven* were entirely cured; *fourteen* were improved, but left before the cure was completed; *six* had suffered such organic changes as to be incurable, though symptoms were palliated.

Only three out of the one hundred and thirty-five cases required the operation of a daily replacement of the uterus. And yet, had I pursued the methods of the practitioners referred to, probably nearly one hundred of my patients would have received this very trying, and, in most cases, needless treatment.   This is stated for the special consideration, not only of patients, but of those practitioners who, like myself, have been led to try the methods of those who, however great their success, owed none of it to *this part* of their treatment.   This subject is important, not only in its *medical* but its *moral* aspect.

[In reference to the dangers here intimated, it is important that the public should be generally apprised of the fact that these and *other* objectionable methods have been introduced both into health establishments and private practice.   At the same time, every woman should be cautioned not to submit to any kind of medical treatment for this class of diseases, which is a *secret* withheld from the profession, nor till she has the assurance of *more than one* physician that the method proposed is indispensable to her relief from great suffering.—C. E. B.]

3. *Symptoms of Pelvic Displacement, and their Treatment.*

The fact that the development of this particular form of disease among women, until lately, has been rare, and that there has been but little popular published information on the subject, has led to other incidental evils which need to be noticed.

The pelvic organs are subject to a great variety of displacements, and of functional and organic diseases.   And yet they all have so many symptoms in common, that it requires not only good anatomical, pathological, and physiological knowledge, but close and well-cultivated diagnostic powers to decide *which* organ is diseased, and *how* it is diseased. For example, sometimes a displacement of the uterus will cause a sense of weight, dragging, and throbbing, accompanied by pain in the back and in front of the hips. But inflammation, ulceration, and induration of this organ will produce precisely the same results; and sometimes *mere nervous debility* in these parts will induce these symptoms, especially when the imagination is excited in reference to the subject. It also is often the case that extreme prolapsus occurs *in which there is no pain at all.*

So also diseases of the urinary cyst are indicated by symptoms precisely similar to those which mark the disease of the adjacent organ. These organs lying in close proximity, and supplied with nerves from the same source, would necessarily sympathize, and show disease by similar symptoms. Just as in the toothache, many a one has been unable to point out the diseased tooth. How much more difficulty exists in a case where most women are profoundly ignorant on the subject!

It has become a very common notion, that when any local displacement of the pelvic organs occur, a woman must cease to use her arms, cease to exercise vigorously, and keep herself on the bed much of her time. All which, in most cases, is exactly the three things which she ought not to do. And thus it is that, when from want of fresh air and exercise, and from the many pernicious practices that debilitate the female constitution, the pelvic organs indicate debility, and these nerves begin to ache, immediately a harness is put on for local support, and the bed becomes the constant resort. And thus the muscular debility and nervous irritability are increased. And yet, all that is needed is fresh air, exercise, simple diet, and *proper* mental occupation.

In this condition, perhaps, resort is had to some ignorant or inexperienced practitioner, who has some patent supporter to sell, or who has some secret and wonderful method of curing such diseases. Then commences, in many cases, a kind of local treatment most trying to the feelings, *which is but seldom required,* and which, in a majority of cases, results in no benefit.

Many a one has recited to me the mental and physical suffering she has endured for months, in such a course of treatment, and all to no purpose. A touching case of this kind recently occurred, in the case of a beautiful young lady, who was a listener to a course of lectures on the pelvis and its diseases, given by me to the graduating class of a female seminary. At the close, she came to me, and with tearful eyes and a quivering lip, she said, "I see now why all I have suffered in body and mind from my physician is worse than useless. I see now that I have never had the disease for which I have been treated. Is it not shocking that I should have suffered what was so needless, when my physician did or ought to have known better?"

Woman's trusting, confiding nature is beautiful; but oh! how much it needs to be protected by an intelligence on such subjects, that will enable her properly to exercise her own judgment! And surely in such cases, above all others, a woman should be sure that her medical adviser has had a proper education, and possesses a well-established moral character.

4. *Effects of Imagination in reference to these Diseases.*

Besides the evils of misunderstanding and mistreating these affections, we have a host of evils from the effects of imagination. Multitudes of women, who hear terrific accounts of the nature of these complaints, and of the treatment that is inevitable, have their imagination so excited that aches and pains that are really trifling become magnified into all the symptoms of the dreaded evil. They betake themselves to bed, become more and more nervous as they give up air, exercise, and occupation; and thus drag out a useless life, a burden to themselves and to their families. Again and again, I have had such cases brought to me, where for years they could not leave their beds or walk at all, when I had nothing to do but make them understand their own organism, and convince them that they needed little else except to get up and go to work in order to be

O

healthy women. It is such cases that furnish a large portion of the "wonderful cures" that attract patients into the hands of some poorly-qualified practitioners.

It is probable that thousands of women who are suffering from pain in the back and pelvic evils, and who either will soon be invalids or imagine themselves so, could be relieved entirely by obeying these directions:

1. Wash the whole person on rising in cool water. Dress loosely, and let *all* the weight of clothing rest on the shoulders.

2. Sleep in a well-ventilated room; exercise the muscles a great deal, especially those of the arms and trunk, taking care to lie down and rest as soon as fatigue is felt.

3. Take a sitting-bath ten minutes at a time, in the middle of the forenoon and afternoon, with water at 85, reducing it gradually each day till at 60. Let the water reach above the hip, and while bathing rub and press the abdomen *upward*.

Wear a wet double girdle by night around the lower part of the body. Make it one-third of a yard wide; wring it well, and when on, cover it with double cotton flannel. If pain and weakness are felt, wear it by day also, adding clothing enough to prevent chilliness.

5. *Effects of these Complaints on Character and Domestic Happiness.*

My heart aches when I see how the mass of women, by ignorance and by blind bondage to custom and fashion, bring on themselves pangs innumerable and premature old age. Many a blooming bride at twenty, finds herself, at thirty, wrinkled and care-worn; unhappy as a wife, unreasonable as a mother, and almost useless as a citizen. While some have inherited too much physical depravity to be preserved by any methods in good health, the majority have been most miserably spendthrift in using up their vital powers, thus rendering the joy of their married life as evanescent as the morning cloud. Many a wife who, but for her physical condition, would have been happy in her social relation, says to me, with a sigh, "I ought never to have been married, for my life is one prolonged agony.

I could endure it myself alone, but the thought that I am, from year to year, becoming the mother of those who are to partake of and perpetuate the misery that I endure, makes me so wretched that I am well-nigh distracted.

A wife of more than ordinary intelligence and attainments, who had, during the ten years of her married life, been suffering from these evils, asked me, after I had examined her case, if I thought it curable. I told her she could be made more comfortable, but such organic changes *could never be cured.* She burst into tears, and said, 'Oh, that I might die then!" I asked if she was weary of life? She said, "No, it is not on my own account, but my condition is such a trial to my husband; I wish I could give him freedom by taking rest to myself in the grave."

The young miss who wickedly wastes her health, and receives with an indifferent toss of the head all cautions in regard to health, little dreams of the bitter tears she will shed when it is too late for repentance to avail. The prospective husband may take great care to protect the fair but frail one of his choice; he may in after years fondly cherish the wife of his youth when she aches constantly and fades prematurely; still he has no helpmate—no one to double life's joys or lighten life's labors for him. Some sick women grow selfish and forget that, in a partnership such as theirs, others suffer when they suffer. Every true husband has but half a life who has a sick wife.

A few days since a gentleman living with his third wife, whom he had just placed under my care, said, "There is nothing that I have so much desired as a companion *in good health*; but it is what I have seldom enjoyed in all my married life." Then, with a sigh, he rose, and walked quickly to and fro in his spacious parlors, saying, "my home is again shaded by sickness and sorrow, and my last hope of domestic joy is blighted." His elegant residence and political honors could give him no enjoyment while his wife was an invalid.

A young husband, in thriving business, of naturally a hopeful heart, presents the case of his wife, and asks, "Can she ever be well? Will she ever have her former hopeful, loving, patient spirit ?" Then the tears gathered as he said, "We used to be happy, but now, when I come from business, she can only tell of her suffering, and reproach me because I do not try more to relieve her." Then he added, by way of self-defense, "I do try to nurse her, and tend baby when I can be spared from business; I get the best help I can, but nothing satisfies—*she is so nervous!*" The wife, I found, had been brought up elegantly but indolently, and so neither body nor spirit were developed sufficiently to bear healthfully the changes which maternity induces.

There are no class of infirmities more likely to induce irritability of temper and depression of spirit than those that affect the pelvic organs. A husband, whose wife had spent some months with us as a patient, said afterward that he should consider her stay there the best investment he ever made, even if there had been no other improvement in his wife than the change in her temper.

6. *Peculiar Instruction needed by young Children*

Through information gained from my husband, from other physicians, from teachers, from medical writers, and from the reports of insane hospitals, it has become clear to my mind that there are secret and terrific causes preying extensively upon the health and nervous energy of childhood and youth of both sexes, such as did not formerly exist, and such as demand new efforts to eradicate and prevent.

Parents and teachers all over the land need to be made aware that a secret vice is becoming frequent among children of both sexes, that is taught by servants and communicated by children at school. Indeed, it may result from accident or disease, with an innocent unconsciousness of the evil done, on the part of the child, while the practice may thus ignorantly be perpetuated to maturity. This practice leads to diseases of the most horrible description, to mania, and to fatuity. Death and the mad-house are the last resort of these most miserable victims.

To protect childhood and youth from this, it is not only needful to cultivate purity of mind and personal modesty, but to teach them, while quite young, that any fingering of the parts referred to involves terrible penalties. No such explicit information should be given as would tempt the incautious curiosity of childhood, but the child should be impressed with a sense of guilt and awful punishment as connected with *any thing* of this kind, that would instantly recur to mind if led by accident or instruction to this vice.

In regard to those who have already become victims, to a greater or less degree, to this vice, one caution is very important. Medical writers and others who have attempted to guard the young in this direction, have painted not only the danger but the wickedness of this practice, in such strong colors that, when a young person first discovers the nature of a practice that has been indulged with little conception of the danger or wrong, overaction on the fears and the conscience is not unfrequently the result. Such horror and despair sometimes ensue as almost paralyze any effort on the part of medical advisers to remedy the evil.

In all such cases, it is safest and best to assume that the sin is one of ignorance, and that the cure is almost certain if the directions given are strictly obeyed. Unstimulating diet, a great deal of exercise in the open air, daily ablution of the whole person, control of the imagination, and occupation of the mind in useful pursuits, will usually remedy the evil after its nature is understood.

In reference to *social*, as well as secret vices of this description, it seems to me the protection of ignorance should be preserved as long as possible, and yet, so that when such knowledge dawns, there shall immediately recur the needful impression of danger and sin. These duties belong especially to parents and teachers; and the circulation of books and papers, with the gross and pernicious information that many have recommended and practiced, involves, as it seems to me, most hazardous results.

[A lady, after reading the above, stated that within the last year a little boy under her care, of very delicate mind and susceptible temperament, was sent to the country to a private boarding-school, under the care of a most excellent gentleman and his wife, who were eminently faithful so far as they knew how to be. The child stayed only six weeks, and returned sick, depressed, and with a burden on his mind that could not be discovered. After learning that he would not be sent back, he revealed the shocking story, and also the fact that the boys had threatened to kill him if he ever told any one.

Another lady, after reading this article, related a similar story of a large and highly respected boarding-school for boys, and gave several mournful incidents to show the effects of such evils on the health of the pupils. Parents whose young sons are at boarding-schools *can not* be too much alarmed on this subject.]

7. *Instructions at a more mature Age.*

You wish my views and experience in reference to instructions that should be communicated to the young on such topics at a more mature age.

The terrible effects I have seen from *simple ignorance*, both on individual and domestic happiness, convince me that a great work is to be attempted in this direction. More than half the cases of extreme suffering which have come under my care, could have been saved had the course that is aimed at by you and your associates have been secured by them. I have been called repeatedly to lecture to young ladies near the close of a school-education, on subjects so important to their future health and happiness, and I never found the least difficulty either on their part or my own.

When the proper discriminations are made between *true* delicacy and propriety, and a fastidious and mawkish imitation of them, there is no difficulty in making them understood and appreciated. I have found, on such occasions, if a person was present known to be wanting in purity and delicacy, it was such only who made very offensive protestations against the course pursued in such instructions.

I believe that the method proposed by your Association of securing by endowments well-qualified ladies, whose *official* duty it shall be to train the young to be healthy, and to communicate all the knowledge that will fit them to fulfill healthfully and happily all their future duties and relations, will, so far as it is carried out, effectually remedy the evils, and secure the benefits designed.

8. *Deterioration of American Women.*

It is impossible for me to communicate in any form suitable to present to the public the views I have expressed (and which all who practice in the departments that bring our sex into special treatment share in common) on one important subject, *i. e.* the deterioration of American women in all the functions connected with maternity. I can only indicate some considerations and facts that perhaps may suggest the most important ideas.

In the pages you read to me on the brain and its laws of health, it is seen that there may be such excesses, even in lawful enjoyments and lawful duties as eventually to exhaust the fountain of nervous energy. In other cases excesses may exhaust the supply in *certain* directions, while in other directions the overworked organs may become habitually and unhealthfully excited.

In reference to this law of physiology, we find three classes of women. The first are those whose brain and nervous system have been so equably and healthily developed that every moral, intellectual, social, domestic, and physical operation is carried on *equably, appropriately,* and *happily.* Every duty is so connected with pleasure, that life is a united, harmonious succession of duties and enjoyments. Such women are becoming, like angel visitants, "few and far between."

The second class are those whose brain and nervous system have been so severely taxed, either by excessive intellectual developments unbalanced by proper exercise; or by excessive labor without amusements; or by excessive pleasure-seeking, and indulgence in various sensitive gratifications, that the nervous fountain is exhausted; so that when the duties connected with maternity commence, almost every thing is wrong, and almost every thing is wanting which a bounteous Creator designed should bless the most sacred relations of life.

The third class are those whose sensitive nature and imagination have been precociously developed in such a course as wealth and indulgence secures. These become morbidly sensitive in dangerous directions, and sometimes

O

the victims of secret or social vices that prey on both character and life.

Oh, that all parents who are to train the *next* generation could be made to understand these intimations, and save their daughters from the abounding anguish which has come upon such multitudes of those now upon the stage!

Very truly yours,   R. B. GLEASON.

NOTE II.

OF the health establishments known to the author, there are two which the author believes to be freest from the defects, and to combine the most advantages indicated in the letter on this topic. These are the one at Elmira, New York, under the care of Dr. and Mrs. Gleason; the other is at Clifton, New York, under the care of Dr. Foster. The chief reason, however, for the selection, is the fact that a well-educated female physician in both these establishments will have the charge of that class of diseases which most appropriately are treated by women.

THERE are two works on Domestic Economy by the writer which have had a wide circulation for many years. The first is named "A Treatise on Domestic Economy." It was prepared as a text-book for schools, and has been extensively used for this purpose. It contains minute instructions in regard to all departments of domestic economy. These were derived not only from personal experience but from the observation and contributions of many of the best housekeepers in the nation.

The second work is called "The Domestic Receipt Book." It aims to teach all that appertains to the care and preparation of food for a family, and provides a great variety of receipts in all departments of cookery.

While, in order to secure a sale of the last book, it was necessary to embrace many receipts that are in violation of those laws of health which are set forth in the volume itself, the evil it was hoped would be met by the instructions given, and by an abundance of receipts for simple and healthful food.

After October, 1855, this Receipt Book will be presented in an improved form, and contain many additional receipts for a great variety of simple and healthful food. Orders may be sent to me for these works also, as directed at page 192, and they will be sent by mail at the same price as at book stores, which is 75 cents a volume. Postage stamps can be used to make change where even dollars are not remitted.

All the net profits on books thus ordered will be paid to the Benevolent Association, and the amount published in their Annual Report.

NOTE IV.

In addition to the immediate practical point in hand, it is possible that my opportunities of investigation in regard to animal magnetism and its kindred manifestations, may enable me to contribute something toward a better understanding of these subjects.

At a very early period in my experience, I arrived at a *theory*, which I will first state and then give some portions of my observations as illustrating it.

The nervous fluid is generated in the brain by our *will*, and can be directed by the will to different portions of the brain and nervous system. It can also be thus directed to the brain and nervous system of *other* persons by mesmeric passes. By this process, the fluid sent forth from the magnetizer accumulates in the brain of the magnetized person, very much as electricity accumulates in a Leyden jar.

In this condition, the magnetized person has the intellectual powers considerably stimulated, and certain new powers brought into action, which are *abnormal*. Opium and alcohol, ether and chloroform, produce similar exaltations.

When the brain is thus excited by an excess of nervous fluid, it becomes highly sensitive to a magnetic or electric fluid that *pervades all space*, and, by this means, the brain comes into the same relation to this medium as the eye holds to *light*. That is, in this state, the mind *perceives*, by the instrumentality of this all-pervading medium, as through the eye it perceives by means of light.

In this state also, the brain of the magnetized person becomes so united, by this medium, to the brains of other persons, especially to that of the magnetizer, as to have access to the knowledge and memory of other minds. Thus, aided and guided by the will of the person who is in magnetic connection, the clairvoyant can *see with the brain* by the aid of this pervading medium, and, to a certain extent, can come into connection with other places and other brains at great distances.

In this state, also, the magnetizer has a certain power over the intellectual faculties, the senses, and the susceptibilities of the magnetized person, so that, by an act of will, he can stimulate any one of them. Thus he can not only make the subject see, feel, taste, and smell whatever he chooses, but can regulate his intellectual *opinions* and *belief* so long as the magnetic influence remains. This power, in certain cases, can be exerted over the subject *at great distances*.

This nervous fluid can also be sent from the brain of one or more persons into *inanimate objects*, and, after a certain accumulation, these objects become animated, for the time being, and more or less subject to the will of the person who most freely imparts the magnetizing fluid. In this way, chairs and tables can be made to move about, *to spell*, and perform other apparently intelligent actions.

In this condition, the brains of the persons who regulate these developments often act on the inanimate objects while the owner is *unconscious* of the operation his brain is performing.

I will now illustrate the several points of this theory, by some portions of my own observation.

Early in December, 1844, having heard, through most reliable persons, of the performances of a clairvoyant woman in Boston, I wrote to my family friends ·in various States, East and West, that I should go to that city on the 23d day of that month, and visit this woman between the hours of 9 and 12 A.M.; and I requested them all to note down what they were doing at that time, and also to write a sentence and lay it on the mantle-shelf of their sitting-rooms.

I went on that day, no person in the city knowing that I was to be there. I went from the cars to this woman, whom I had never seen. None of her family knew me or I them, and I did not give my name. She was put in the clairvoyant state, and then I was left alone with her.

I will first narrate what seems to prove that the clairvoyant could actually *see with her brain* by the aid of the fluid that fills all space. I will narrate the conversation just as I remember it, guided by full notes taken the same day.

Miss B. "I want you to go to a friend's house in Hartford." [I mentioned no name.]

Clairvoyant. "Yes, I am there."

Miss B. "I will tell you where to go."

C. "No—I know where. It is a large white house, set back from the road, not far from a large Asylum."

Miss B. "Has it pillars?"

C. "Yes."

Miss B. "Count them."

C. "Eight."

Miss B. "Go in, and tell me what you see.

C. "Why, what a big entry! It looks like all the house!"

Miss B. "What sort of doors are there, and how many?"

C. "There are four, and two folding-doors. The doors are black; I don't like them. Here is a piano in this entry, and a young girl, with darkish complexion, playing on it."

Miss B. "Who is in the parlor?"

C. "Here is a small, elderly woman. She has a cap on. She has dark complexion and dark eyes. She is reading a book about somebody. She says she don't like it. There is a tall lady there. She is your sister. Is there somebody here named Mary? I hear some one say Mary. The little woman is not well. She thinks she has water on her chest. Her heart troubles her. Her feet swell, and she has to bandage them. Your sister is now in the room where they eat, washing something that looks like a large bowl; it shines. Here is a great Newfoundland dog. I am afraid of him. He jumps up on to me. Will he hurt me?"

Miss B. "Now go into the other parlor."

C. "This room is dark. The shutters are all closed, but I can open one. They won't like it, I suppose, but I don't care. Here is a picture over the fireplace. The hair is brushed up. It looks like your father, only younger. May be it is one of his sons. There is a large picture on the floor."

Miss B. " What sort of a picture ?"

C. " Oh, it is a beautiful, large landscape. It has a great many trees on it. It looks pleasant there under the trees." [This picture always hung in another room, and was set there after I left. She described it as out of its ordinary place, and yet so that I recognized it immediately.]

Now in this case, the lady who was ill supposed she had the affections described; though I had never known it, nor any other person except her physician. She was reading such a book, and did express that opinion of it. My sister was in the room where they ate, washing a large lamp-shade. And these, and many other as minute particulars that I could not have known, were exactly correct, and *she made no mistakes.* It must be remembered, too, that the clairvoyant did not know me, and I never told her the name of the person to whose house I wished her to go.

I asked her how she knew where to go. Her reply was, " I go with your mind to the place, and then I see for myself."

The following illustrates the fact that the clairvoyant had such a connection with my brain that my knowledge and memory were at her command:

Miss B. " I want you to go to Cincinnati."

C. " Yes, I am there. What a beautiful city this is ! I never was here before. They have handsome churches here."

Miss B. " I want you to go to a friend's house in that city. The house has an iron fence in front."

" *C.* Yes, I see it. It has pillars in front. It is down in a deep narrow yard. The people are in the back parlor. There are some children here. One little girl has dark complexion and dark eyes. Another is very fair, has blue eyes and light-colored curls. She is very pretty, and is playing with something. These people are pretty well off. They have got sofas enough I hope. Here are two in this room, and one in the other, and a large, handsome, stuffed chair. There are some handsome pictures here. One is a picture of a gentleman with white hair. It is your uncle. There is a picture of a little girl, with a dog by her, and her hat on the ground. How well that dog's nose is painted !"

In this case the clairvoyant described the room to me exactly as it was, *when I was last there*, but not as it really was at this time, when it was shut up, and the furniture changed. The exclamation about the dog was one I often had made, and heard others make.

But the most striking incident in this case was the following. These friends had lost an only son, *named George*. Recently an infant had arrived, but I had not learned any other particulars. I had written to these friends, to write something and put it on the mantle-shelf of their sitting-room. After many other particulars in regard to the people, house, and furniture had been remarked upon by the clairvoyant, she went on thus:

"There is a baby up stairs. It is a boy. It is asleep, and a girl is taking care of it. This chamber has *queer windows*. They are small and *square*. What do people make such windows for?"

I then asked her to look on the mantle-shelf below, and see if there was a paper with writing on it. She then continued thus: "There is some writing pinned to the wall over the mantle. It is too small. It ought to be written larger. You told them to do this. The first words are—' *The baby's name is*—' I can not read it, it is too small."

"*Try!*" said I, with greatly excited interest. She grasped her hands tightly together, and shook all over, as if making a great effort. Then she said, "Yes, I see it. It is written, ' *The baby's name is George.*'"

Now every minute particular as to the people, house, and furniture corresponded with my past experience. But this matter about the writing was all concocted by herself from materials in my past knowledge. For the baby's name was not George, and there was no paper prepared as I had requested. Nor was I conscious of thinking that the child, if a boy, would be called George after the child that was dead. Indeed, I should not have supposed that this would be the case.

In regard to the papers prepared in other places, she read one aright, though she put it in the wrong family. But in all cases, what she said was written on the papers was appropriate to the persons and place. It was what, from my past knowledge and experience, I might have conjectured would be written.

I had been told by her husband, when he put her into the magnetic sleep, that, *before she was tired*, she would see things as they were, but afterward would see them as I *imagined* them to be. This seemed to be the fact, with the addition, that she made new combinations of her own.

She told me she could see best in a cold, clear, dry day, which are just the circumstances in which an electric machine works the most perfectly.

I visited her at three different times. The two first times she was very clear and correct, always describing things either as they actually were, or consistently with my past experience. The third time she made many mistakes, but she told me beforehand that she was not as well as usual, and that she could not do as she did before.

She did not wait for questions, and seemed impatient when first I attempted to guide or help her.

I took her to nine different places, and, on the first two days, I could not puzzle her or make her describe any thing different from what was either the reality, or my conception of it, or new combinations furnished by my past experience.

But this case shows that no reliance can be placed on the descriptions of clairvoyants. For no one can say when it is that they see things as they are, or when they are using materials furnished by the minds of those connected with them—*ad libitum.*

The next case is one in which I witnessed the phenomena of what is called *psychology*, in which the magnetizer has control of the *senses*, *intellect*, and *belief*.

In this case I saw a large number of persons all magnetized at once, by simply holding a piece of silver in the hand and gazing fixedly at it, while the magnetizer exerted his influence. Of the persons affected in this way, two were respectable mature gentlemen of my brother's church, very quiet, modest men, who in their right minds could never be induced to such performances in any circumstances, much less in public. I saw them at the direction of the magnetizer walk on to an elevated stage, and perform various ridiculous grimaces and contortions for a considerable length of time.   I saw others made to believe that they were scalded by some cold water, which the magnetizer made them, by his word, believe was boiling water.   They screamed and acted just as one does when scalded.   Many other deceptions were practiced thus, and upon persons whose testimony was perfectly reliable.

These performances I have encountered in various quarters, and have heard the most intelligent and reliable persons relate their own experience and that of others so often that it seems to me that such performances can be established by an almost endless amount of reliable evidence.   I have seen persons who were made to believe themselves other men, and to adopt political or religious opinions to which they were in their natural state opposed, and for several consecutive hours till the magnetic fluid passed off.

I have also seen persons who in their natural state possessed a magnetic sensibility similar to that of a clairvoyant in this respect, that after fixing their attention earnestly upon me for some time, they would be conscious of a train of thought which was a reproduction of some periods in my past experience.   I have also read well-authenticated cases of the same nature.

One of my family friends, in a very reduced state of health, became so susceptible to the magnetic influence that one of my brothers, without putting her in the magnetic sleep, could move her head and arms by his will as he did his own.

During this period she seemed to pass into the invisible world, to converse with departed friends, and to realize all her *previous conceptions*, but gained no new ideas.   The memory of this lasted for months as a reality.

I will now narrate some of my observations of the " *spirit rapping*" agency.

I have repeatedly been in families where some of the members had the power of imparting their own nervous fluid to articles of furniture and then making them move, spell, and play various pranks.

I have seen a mahogany table hanging by the hands of persons entirely unsupported by any thing except the hands *held over it*.

I have seen a table without castors and on a carpet, move around the room with me on it, and no other motive power except the will of a lady whose hands rested lightly on the top.

I have seen a large table dance to the sound of a violin in ways which I am sure no man or men, by any ordinary method, could produce, while no motive power was visible except the hands of certain persons laid lightly on the top.

I have seen friends who were perfectly reliable take a pencil in the left hand and put it behind them and thus write sentences in a foreign language, while they assured me they had not the least conception of what was thus produced.

And I have seen multitudes of persons of perfectly good sense and credibility relate similar and still more remarkable performances.

In all this I have never seen any good reason for inferring any other agency but that of *a newly-discovered method of employing the nervous fluid generated in the human brain, and acting in connection with the pervading medium that fills all space.*

On this subject there are three maxims of common sense to guide us.

The first is, that we are to rely on the testimony of our own senses, except when we have evidence that they are diseased or disordered.

The next is, that we are to rely on human testimony when those testifying have full opportunity to judge, are credible persons, and have no motive to deceive.

The third is, that we are not to infer any supernatural agencies for effects that *can* be accounted for without any such inference.

Such facts as I have here narrated have been proved by an abundance of testimony from credible persons as what has again and again been tested by their senses, while there was no motive to tempt them to deceive. And if all this evidence and testimony may be set aside, how are we to establish the miracles on which Christianity rests?

The attempt to do this is an attempt that directly tends to undermine faith in the Bible.

But all difficulties are avoided by discriminating between

the facts proved and the *theory* by which we account for these facts. We may adopt the facts as true and yet refuse a theory which is deemed false and pernicious.

It has seemed to me that instead of fearing to examine and believe in the reality of the facts of magnetism and clairvoyance, as here set forth, that the safe course is in the opposite direction. For whether they are established or not, they are a most powerful *argument ad hominem* against those who uphold the interference of disembodied spirits in the spirit rapping demonstration.

For they concede that persons can be in the clairvoyant state *while awake* and possessing other ordinary power, and that in this state the mind of the clairvoyant has access to places at great distances, and to the memory and knowledge of other minds in any place where it ranges. At the same time, it is seen that articles of furniture can be so filled with the nervous fluid as to be moved by human volitions and thus be made to spell by knocks and other movements. Moreover, I have myself seen cases where the ideas of my own brain were reproduced in another mind, while this mind, guided in a measure by mine, brought out new and yet consistent combinations of the materials my past experience provided. And it was done *without any consciousness on my part of willing it.* An example of this is seen in the case where the clairvoyant spelled the name of the child, and in the cases where she told what was written on the papers. In all these cases she was guided by my will to look for papers and to read what was on them, while she manufactured her results from my past knowledge, without any action of my will so far as I could judge.

If, then, the abnormal accumulation of the nervous fluid in the brain, and in articles of furniture, can impart such powers, it furnishes data sufficient to account for all the phenomena claimed to result from the agency of disembodied spirits without resorting to this agency as a cause.

And of course we are required in this, as in all other matters, to apply the rule of common sense, that we are not to infer any supernatural agencies for effects that can be accounted for without any such inference.

I have as yet never seen any thing claimed to be " spiritual manifestations" that could not be easily accounted for as is here suggested.   And the progress of time is more and more exhibiting the folly and inconsistency of the popular delusion that brings back the spirits of departed friends to perform fantastic tricks, and to make known inane and contradictory revelations.

The whole matter of animal magnetism and its kindred associates, as they have been developed to me, seem to involve an unnatural and abnormal action on the human system which is dangerous, liable to great perversions, and redeemed by little that is healthful or remedial.

Many facts that have come to my knowledge within a few months, have convinced me that no woman should submit to the influence of magnetic power except in great emergencies, and then only with great care and precaution.

Note V.

FRONT AND BACK VIEW OF THE HUMAN SKELETON.

Fig. 1.

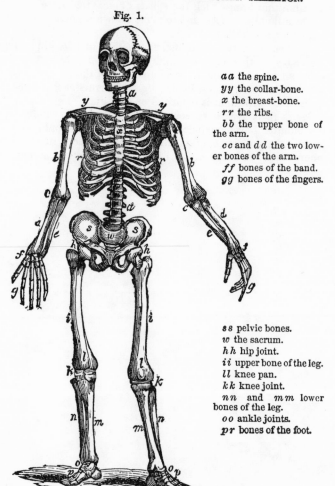

a a the spine.
y y the collar-bone.
x the breast-bone.
r r the ribs.
b b the upper bone of the arm.
c c and *d d* the two lower bones of the arm.
f f bones of the hand.
g g bones of the fingers.

s s pelvic bones.
w the sacrum.
h h hip joint.
i i upper bone of the leg.
l l knee pan.
k k knee joint.
n n and *m m* lower bones of the leg.
o o ankle joints.
p r bones of the foot.

Front View of the Skeleton.

Fig. 2.

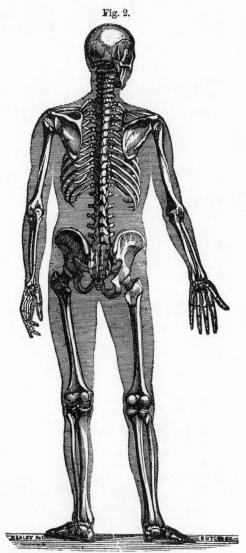

Rear View of the Skeleton.

Medicine & Society In America

An Arno Press/New York Times Collection

Alcott, William A. **The Physiology of Marriage.** 1866. New Introduction by Charles E. Rosenberg.

Beard, George M. **American Nervousness: Its Causes and Consequences.** 1881. New Introduction by Charles E. Rosenberg.

Beard, George M. **Sexual Neurasthenia.** 5th edition. 1898.

Beecher, Catharine E. **Letters to the People on Health and Happiness.** 1855.

Blackwell, Elizabeth. **Essays in Medical Sociology.** 1902. Two volumes in one.

Blanton, Wyndham B. **Medicine in Virginia in the Seventeenth Century.** 1930.

Bowditch, Henry I. **Public Hygiene in America.** 1877.

Bowditch, N[athaniel] I. **A History of the Massachusetts General Hospital:** To August 5, 1851. 2nd edition. 1872.

Brill, A. A. **Psychanalysis: Its Theories and Practical Application.** 1913.

Cabot, Richard C. **Social Work:** Essays on the Meeting-Ground of Doctor and Social Worker. 1919.

Cathell, D. W. **The Physician Himself and What He Should Add to His Scientific Acquirements.** 2nd edition. 1882. New Introduction by Charles E. Rosenberg.

The Cholera Bulletin. Conducted by an Association of Physicians. Vol. I: Nos. 1–24. 1832. All published. New Introduction by Charles E. Rosenberg.

Clarke, Edward H. **Sex in Education;** or, A Fair Chance for the Girls. 1873.

Committee on the Costs of Medical Care. **Medical Care for the American People:** The Final Report of The Committee on the Costs of Medical Care, No. 28. [1932].

Currie, William. **An Historical Account of the Climates and Diseases of the United States of America.** 1792.

Davenport, Charles Benedict. **Heredity in Relation to Eugenics.** 1911. New Introduction by Charles E. Rosenberg.

Davis, Michael M. **Paying Your Sickness Bills.** 1931.

Disease and Society in Provincial Massachusetts: Collected Accounts, 1736–1939. 1972.

Earle, Pliny. **The Curability of Insanity:** A Series of Studies. 1887.

Falk, I. S., C. Rufus Rorem, and Martha D. Ring. **The Costs of Medical Care:** A Summary of Investigations on The Economic Aspects of the Prevention and Care of Illness, No. 27. 1933.

Faust, Bernhard C. **Catechism of Health:** For the Use of Schools, and for Domestic Instruction. 1794.

Flexner, Abraham. **Medical Education in the United States and Canada:** A Report to The Carnegie Foundation for the Advancement of Teaching, Bulletin Number Four. 1910.

Gross, Samuel D. **Autobiography of Samuel D. Gross, M.D.,** with Sketches of His Contemporaries. Two volumes. 1887.

Hooker, Worthington. **Physician and Patient;** or, A Practical View of the Mutual Duties, Relations and Interests of the Medical Profession and the Community. 1849.

Howe, S. G. **On the Causes of Idiocy.** 1858.

Jackson, James. **A Memoir of James Jackson, Jr., M.D.** 1835.

Jennings, Samuel K. **The Married Lady's Companion, or Poor Man's Friend.** 2nd edition. 1808.

The Maternal Physician; a Treatise on the Nurture and Management of Infants, from the Birth until Two Years Old. 2nd edition. 1818. New Introduction by Charles E. Rosenberg.

Mathews, Joseph McDowell. **How to Succeed in the Practice of Medicine.** 1905.

McCready, Benjamin W. **On the Influences of Trades, Professions, and Occupations in the United States, in the Production of Disease.** 1943.

Mitchell, S. Weir. **Doctor and Patient.** 1888.

Nichols, T[homas] L. **Esoteric Anthropology:** The Mysteries of Man. [1853].

Origins of Public Health in America: Selected Essays, 1820–1855. 1972.

Osler, Sir William. **The Evolution of Modern Medicine.** 1922.

The Physician and Child-Rearing: Two Guides, 1809–1894. 1972.

Rosen, George. **The Specialization of Medicine:** with Particular Reference to Ophthalmology. 1944.

Royce, Samuel. **Deterioration and Race Education.** 1878.

Rush, Benjamin. **Medical Inquiries and Observations.** Four volumes in two. 4th edition. 1815.

Shattuck, Lemuel, Nathaniel P. Banks, Jr., and Jehiel Abbott. **Report of a General Plan for the Promotion of Public and Personal Health.** Massachusetts Sanitary Commission. 1850.

Smith, Stephen. **Doctor in Medicine** and Other Papers on Professional Subjects. 1872.

Still, Andrew T. **Autobiography of Andrew T. Still,** with a History of the Discovery and Development of the Science of Osteopathy. 1897.

Storer, Horatio Robinson. **The Causation, Course, and Treatment of Reflex Insanity in Women.** 1871.

Sydenstricker, Edgar. **Health and Environment.** 1933.

Thomson, Samuel. **A Narrative, of the Life and Medical Discoveries of Samuel Thomson.** 1822.

Ticknor, Caleb. **The Philosophy of Living;** or, The Way to Enjoy Life and Its Comforts. 1836.

U.S. Sanitary Commission. **The Sanitary Commission of the United States Army:** A Succinct Narrative of Its Works and Purposes. 1864.

White, William A. **The Principles of Mental Hygiene.** 1917.